KICK THAT MIGRAINE

Mastering the Three Key Concepts
to End Migraines Naturally

Lilli-Marlene Clemens-Stäheli ND

KICK THAT MIGRAINE
Mastering the three key concepts
to end migraines naturally

First published in Australia by Lilli-Marlene Clemens-Stäheli ND 2025
lilliclemens.com

Copyright © Lilli-Marlene Clemens-Stäheli ND 2025
All Rights Reserved

A catalogue record for this
book is available from the
National Library of Australia

ISBN: 978-1-7640852-0-5 (pbk)
ISBN: 978-1-7640852-1-2 (ebk)

Typesetting and design by Publicious Book Publishing
Published in collaboration with Publicious Book Publishing
www.publicious.com.au

'*To nature, whose unwavering wisdom resides in the earth, the plants and the elements, and to the quiet strength of natural healing—unhurried, yet profound.*'

Lilli-Marlene Clemens-Stäheli ND

Table of Contents

Acknowledgments

I would like to express my deepest gratitude to the many patients who have shared with me their stories, struggles and triumphs over the years in my clinic. Your courage, resilience and trust have not only shaped my understanding, but have also inspired the pages of this book. It is through our shared experiences that I have been able to learn, grow and develop the insights that I hope will benefit others.

My heartfelt thanks also go to my sister, Marie-Louise, a kindred spirit and fellow migraine master—celebrating your triumph over migraines. Thank you for the many deep conversations we've shared. Your empathy, insight and support have been a source of immense inspiration.

About the Author

Lilli Clemens-Stäheli is an accomplished naturopath, lecturer and researcher with a strong academic and clinical background. She earned her Bachelor's degree in Naturopathy in 2004 and has since pursued various postgraduate studies, including Nutrition Medicine at the Royal Melbourne Institute of Technology in 2006, and Public Health at Curtin University in 2014. She also obtained a Master's degree in Human Nutrition from Deakin University in 2017. Additionally, Lilli is a certified Pilates instructor, having received her full Pilates instructor certification from Pilates International in 2004.

Over the course of her career, Lilli has gained valuable clinical experience through her work at two busy multi-modality clinics on the Gold Coast, spanning 18 years. Specialising primarily in migraines, Lilli has also contributed to the field of natural health as a practitioner, lecturer and student clinic supervisor. Lilli's multifaceted background in natural health, nutrition and higher education has equipped her with a unique skill set that allows her to excel in her profession and have a meaningful impact on the lives of her clients and students.

Preface

The aim in writing this book was to put my understanding into context and provide an informative insight into the complex and multifaceted causes of the migraine condition. Bridging the gap in understanding migraines is long overdue, not only for patients seeking relief but also for practitioners eager to deepen their knowledge. My aim was to unravel the complex interplay of factors that contribute to migraines and to empower both individuals and professionals with the tools and insights necessary to address this condition effectively.

The accumulation of knowledge from my own personal migraine journey, along with insights gained from the experiences of my many patients, has provided a unique perspective in how natural medicine has the capacity to help master migraines.

The detailed notes, schematics and observations I have gathered over the years have merged into a comprehensive understanding and treatment of this condition. The holistic treatments and strategies in this book have been carefully selected, are evidence-based and have been rigorously used and assessed with patients in my clinic, demonstrating significant benefits.

This book is not just a passive resource; it serves as a portal to a journey of transformation, offering readers the knowledge, insights and practical tools they need to 'kick that migraine'. It has made writing this book a challenge but also an extremely rewarding task.

For some of you, the detailed discussions on chemical and biological processes may feel a bit overwhelming at times. That's completely fine. If you encounter sections that feel too technical, you can choose to skip ahead without losing the essence of the content. At the end of each section, you will find a concise summary in the form of 'brain bites'. These are designed to distil the key points for easier understanding and are paired with actionable strategies you can implement right away.

Remember, this book is meant to be a flexible guide tailored to your needs. Whether you dive deeply into the science or prefer to focus on practical takeaways, there's something here for everyone seeking to better understand and manage migraines. For a more detailed overview of how to navigate this book, I encourage you to read the following section, 'A Roadmap on How to Navigate This Book'. It will provide guidance on how to approach the content to get the most out of every section, ensuring that you understand the core concepts and can apply the strategies to your own journey towards better health.

A roadmap on how to navigate this book
(and some other important morsels to guide you on this journey)

At the heart of this book lies a purposeful mission: to empower you with the knowledge and strategies needed for effective migraine prevention. The book is designed to guide you through three essential concepts that serve as a foundation for understanding and managing migraines. These principles will not only enhance your awareness but also equip you with practical tools to reclaim control over your wellbeing.

The first concept is gaining knowledge, the key for success. Acquiring information and skills is crucial for success in various aspects of life. This approach is equally vital when addressing your migraines. Understanding your own personal migraines and how they develop, will allow you to apply and monitor preventative treatments to successfully reduce their frequency and severity.

The second concept will help you to master your personal triggers and premonition symptoms. You will develop a heightened awareness, and refine your intuition and ability to discern and interpret all those obscure triggers and premonitions. Every person's migraine profile is unique like a fingerprint and by identifying your own specific migraine characteristics, will enable you to take proactive steps in managing your migraines.

The third concept will address the sensitivity factor and restore brain plasticity. This will focus on lowering stress patterns and breaking the inflammatory cycle. You will also learn about your body's vulnerabilities and discover how to restore vitality and resilience by addressing underlying metabolic imbalances and sensitivities.

With these three key concepts in mind, you will find five distinct chapters in this book, each offering a unique perspective and complementing the others, contributing to a holistic understanding of migraines. This will in turn help you to form an essential foundation for success in conquering your migraine. The five chapters are interconnected, yet can be explored independently, creating a dynamic learning experience. Feel free to explore the book in any order that suits your reading style. Whether you prefer a linear approach or want to jump between chapters, the organisation is designed to accommodate your preferences.

Each chapter is organised with section headers that break the content into specific topics. At the end of each section, a summary of key points, referred to as 'brain bites', will guide you to further information, including cross-references to relevant strategies and treatment options, which are navigable by their section numbers.

In the back of this book, you will also find a glossary that provides an explanation of words, or terms that are specific to the content of the book. The glossary is arranged in alphabetical order, making it easy to find the meanings of unfamiliar or specialised terms used within the text.

Lastly, and perhaps most importantly, you will be directed to a practical tool: a migraine diary, which you will learn about in Chapter 5. This personalised health tool will help turn your knowledge into actionable steps and customise your health journey, enabling you to better understand your condition through self-reflection. You can immediately apply what you have learned by using the diary to track your migraine patterns, triggers and symptoms.

I hope these navigation tips make your reading and learning experience smoother. Wishing you all the best in your healing journey.

Now, go and Kick that Migraine!

Staying Committed to your Health Journey

Making changes to health and lifestyle can pose a considerable challenge. While the idea may seem promising in theory, the actual implementation often proves to be more demanding than anticipated. Personally, I experienced the difficulty firsthand, yielding no tangible results. Consequently, it becomes tempting to find all sorts of reasons to abandon the effort altogether. However, it is crucial not to succumb to the belief that the task is impossible, nor should we think that attempting change is futile. As Roy Bennett aptly put it, '*Do not fear failure but rather fear not trying.*'

Making changes from a grassroots approach to health has its personal obstacles and challenges and you will find that in this health journey that you are about to endeavour, it is important to have a positive attitude and focus on progress rather than perfection. Some of the traits that are particularly important to help your success are firstly motivation. Ask yourself what your personal motivation is for making the change and how critical is it for you to succeed. If you have ticked the motivation box, then you need to consider discipline and consistency. Making personal changes and sticking to new routines requires discipline and self-control. This will also include making time for self-care, such as stress-management techniques and recording information in your daily trigger diary.

With motivation and discipline comes patience. Changing health and lifestyle takes time and will not happen overnight. From a natural order of things, the body needs time to heal and adapt.

It's important to have patience and persistence in the face of setbacks and to celebrate small victories along the way.

Here are some key principles to keep you motivated and on track:

Be Open to Change

- Stay adaptable and willing to try new approaches.

- Be patient with progress as natural medicine often takes time to work. Don't get discouraged if change feels slow. These are subtle changes that address underlying imbalances rather than providing immediate relief. This is a long-term wellness journey.

Listen to Your Body

- Self-awareness and reflecting on your daily habits will help you better understand how your body responds to the environment around you and the changes you make.

- Take time to reflect on your habits and routines and track your progress. Keeping a migraine diary will help you review them and recognise potential patterns.

Set Realistic Goals

- Start small and specific. Remember that knowledge is one of the three keys for success.

- Don't skip important steps in treatment.

- Small, achievable goals can be integrated into daily life more easily, making long-term adherence more likely.

- Achieving small, incremental goals builds confidence and helps you feel empowered in your migraine management journey.

Stay Positive

- Focus on the positives of your journey rather than dwelling on setbacks. A positive mindset can greatly enhance your resilience. Rest can help maintain overall well-being and increase the chances of success in making health and lifestyle changes.

Build a Strong Support System

- Surround yourself with like-minded friends and family, and work with a healthcare practitioner who understands your approach. A strong community can offer emotional support, practical advice and motivation.

'Do not fear failure but rather fear not trying.'
Roy T Bennett

This is My Story

As Hippocrates said, 'Desperate times call for desperate measures', and from my humble beginnings, with little knowledge of migraines, I did just that. I followed the pharmaceutical path to no avail, scouring Google for every possible remedy, trying to determine the cause of my migraines, hoping to find that one solution to conquer them all. In my pursuit of relief, I abstained not only from my beloved red wine but from alcohol altogether, forsaking even the temptation of delectable chocolate. Oh, the sacrifices one makes! If there is such a thing as a 'chocolate gene', I certainly have it.

Additionally, I have learned meditation to reduce stress, joined a yoga class, and adopted a vegan lifestyle to avoid histamines. Determined to improve blood flow to my brain, I even mastered the art of standing on my head for five minutes a day.

By this point in my journey, I had learned more about migraines, yet somehow my confusion only grew.

Still, I can confidently say, 'Been there, done that.' If any part of this story resonates with you, take comfort in knowing you're not alone. Migraines affect about 14% of the global population, making them the third most prevalent disease worldwide.

Fast-forwarding to the present and reflecting on my eighteen years of practice, I have accumulated a substantial body of data from patients and my own experiences with migraines. Over the years, I encountered unforgettable individuals who frequently used vivid and recurring descriptions to convey their migraine experiences. Words like torment, agony, total wretchedness, torture, utter debilitation, and living nightmare came up repeatedly.

One particularly memorable patient was a witty gentleman and stand-up comedian who humorously remarked, 'The English playwright, William Congreve, obviously never suffered from migraines', stating that 'Hell hath no fury like a migraine attack'. Another patient, a middle-aged woman, described her migraines as 'an internal chemical warfare that leaves everything annihilated within.' I am certain many readers can empathise with these sentiments.

My story is not unique. Looking back, I now realise that I experienced two distinct types of migraines. The first was the classic hormonal migraine, occurring with clockwork regularity. In between, I would endure up to three migraines each month. I was prone to stress and dealt with chronic digestive issues and psoriasis. I believe my migraines began with my hormonal cycle at the age of eleven or twelve. In addition to migraines, I frequently suffered from early morning headaches, which occurred as often as four times a week. Typically, one of these episodes would escalate into a full-blown migraine by late morning.

High school marked the onset of frequent migraine episodes. I vividly remember returning home on the school bus, grappling with a splitting headache, accompanied by waves of nausea, hot flushes and beads of sweat trickling down from my armpits. With unwavering determination, I would focus on the passing landscape, determined to avoid the embarrassment of vomiting on the bus.

In my early adulthood, my contemplation of this affliction deepened. The constant apprehension of the impending migraine attacks made me increasingly determined to unravel the root cause of this persistent burdensome health issue.

I was intrigued and puzzled by why some people suffer from migraines while others do not. I discovered that migraines run on both sides of my family, yet very few relatives are affected. Even within my immediate family, only my dad and one of my sisters experience migraines. Nothing seemed to make sense, and I found myself constantly trying to determine what I did differently that led to my migraines.

It wasn't until my doctor mentioned that my migraines had a genetic component and advised me to 'just put up with it'. At the time, I knew little about genes—aside from the fact that *jeans* were my favourite piece of clothing. This marked the beginning of my research journey.

After completing my complementary medical degree, followed by a Masters in human nutrition, I found myself a little wiser in the body's inner workings. At that point, the appeal of gene theory diminished. This doesn't mean I dismiss the importance of genetics, but discussions around genetics often become a common default in mainstream medicine when there are no clear answers to complex conditions.

Nevertheless, our genetic make-up is real, and so are genetic variations, and my perspective has evolved beyond the simplistic notion of a single gene particle bearing the label of 'migraine'. Genetics may indeed play a role in migraine sufferers, but observing the resolution of migraines through natural interventions suggests that it may not be the primary determinant in migraine pathophysiology. Instead, it appears to function as a catalyst, rendering metabolic pathways more susceptible or sensitive to chemical changes.

One way genes may interact is through gene variation. An example is the MTHFR gene, which encodes methylenetetrahydrofolate reductase, an enzyme crucial for regulating the methyl cycle in bodily cells. This gene exists in several variants, and there is much speculation about how these variants may adversely impact the methylation pathway. However, these claims remain largely theoretical, mainly due to the difficulty of scientifically validating the functions of these gene variants. Nevertheless, it is well-established that nutrient deficiencies can greatly influence the methylation process, which should make this the first and foremost approach of treatment.

The functional health of the methylation cycle, along with other biological pathways, is closely tied to epigenetics and represents a valuable area of focus for individuals suffering from migraines. Epigenetics regulates gene expression and is influenced by various factors, including nutrition, lifestyle choices, behaviour, and environmental conditions. Exposure to stress, toxins, inflammation, and nutrient deficiencies can directly alter gene methylation patterns, potentially increasing the risk of developing migraines.

But in all seriousness, with the vast expanse of scientific knowledge at our disposal, I often find myself pondering a pressing question: Why, despite our incredible advancements in so many fields, has there been so little meaningful progress in medicine when it comes to truly improving the quality of life for those who suffer from migraines?

What I discovered is that migraines are far from being a modern affliction. In fact, this condition has been recognised as significant and extraordinary throughout the annals of history. Physicians from ancient civilisations have meticulously documented both the symptoms and the various treatments they employed to alleviate migraines.

The earliest known reference to migraines is found in an ancient Egyptian text called the *Ebers Papyrus*, a medical compendium dating back to around 1550 BC. The papyrus was purchased in Luxor in 1873 by the egyptologist, George Ebers, and is now housed at the University of Leipzig in Germany. Another notable mention of migraines comes from the Greek physician, Hippocrates, who, around 400 BC, described the symptoms of migraines, specifically noting the visual aura that often precedes an attack, as well as various activities that can trigger them. By around 180 AD, the Roman physician, Galen, observed that migraine pain could be alleviated by vomiting, which he believed released an excess of yellow bile from the stomach. Despite the centuries of study, the fact that migraines remain difficult to treat effectively highlights the complexity of this debilitating condition.

Modern medicine has made few significant advancements in migraine treatment; it seems to have reached something of a stalemate. The so-called cutting-edge migraine medications appear to be little more than smoke and mirrors, primarily benefiting the pharmaceutical industries' bottom line rather than the patients who suffer from migraines. Many of the migraine patients I have had the privilege of treating in my clinic had already tried numerous pharmaceutical drugs and various treatments. By the time they arrive at my clinic, their primary concern often revolves around the unsatisfactory outcomes of these medications and the accompanying side effects.

Did you know?
According to a 2020 Google content analysis, there are 77 recommendations
for acute and preventative migraine treatments.[1]

For me, this journey has been exceptionally exciting, drawing from both my clinical experiences and my personal battle with migraines. Even the moments when I subjected myself to my own scientific experiments and endured intense induced migraines have provided me with extraordinary insights into the complex nature of migraine events. Combining my professional observations with my personal experiences has been both challenging and rewarding, significantly enriching my understanding of the complexities surrounding migraines.

I have learned that a purely scientific approach to understanding migraines is greatly limited by the lack of insight from a human encounter. Migraines are not just about chemical pathways and pathology; they also encompass psychological wellbeing, mental and emotional states, and the influence of the surrounding environment. It is not just attempting to inhibit a singular chemical pathway with a singular pharmaceutical chemical, but to restore the body's equilibrium—to understand and address the functional relationships between various body systems, such as the bidirectional interactions between neural and immune responses, metabolic pathways and their connections to the external environment.

This holistic approach recognises that the body operates as an interconnected network, where systems interact and support each other; an imbalance in one area can have cascading effects on overall health. Therefore, interventions must take these intricate interactions into account to promote optimal function and overall wellbeing.

The cause of migraines is not singular but rather a multifaceted interplay of genetic, neurological, environmental, dietary, and hormonal factors, making it a highly individualised condition with varying triggers and manifestations for each person.

Unravelling the cause of migraines is a meticulous process, much like untangling a ball of yarn, working through the knots and complex threads. It is a process that requires observation, determination and diligence in defining and understanding the unique threads contributing to this complex neurological tapestry, which mirrors the complexity but also the beauty of the fundamental biological processes of the human body.

My personal migraine journey has been a long and arduous road, paved with countless tribulations and challenges. It has been a relentless battle, one that demanded unwavering tenacity as I delved deeper into the obscure and complex world of migraine triggers. Each step forward seemed to reveal yet another layer of intricacies, an ever-shifting web of factors that would eventuate to a migraine. The elusive nature of these triggers, with the ability to subtly interact with one another, made each discovery feel both enlightening and vexing.

The more I learned, the more I realised how insidiously migraines could embed themselves in the very fabric of daily life.

At the outset of my journey with migraines, I regarded the migraine diary as a superfluous tool, something I believed would offer little insight. In my mind, the act of jotting down symptoms and experiences felt futile, an exercise in repetition that seemed unlikely to yield any clarity or relief. I dismissed it, thinking that my understanding of my migraines was sufficient without this extra layer of documentation.

However, as time went on, I began to realise that the diary was, in fact, the foundation of my thoughts and reflections. What I once perceived as an unnecessary task, transformed into a valuable compass, guiding me through the complexities of lifestyle and dietary triggers. Each entry became a steppingstone, slowly revealing a formation of recurring patterns. Through careful observation and reflection, it helped me connect the dots between my physical sensations and the complex web of external and internal factors influencing my life and wellbeing. The migraine diary, once deemed needless, evolved into a crucial ally in my endeavour to understand the insights of my personal migraines.

One of the things the migraine diary helped me identify was my most significant triggers. These included stress, hormonal fluctuations during my menstrual cycle, and a number of certain foods, which I had to avoid meticulously. I was particularly susceptible to chocolate and alcoholic beverages, with red wine, port and sherry at the top of the list. Some processed meats, especially ham, bacon and prosciutto, as well as citrus fruits, also played a significant role in my dietary restrictions.

The migraine diary also helped me discover obscure triggers I previously could not pinpoint, giving me a significant advantage in avoiding waking headaches and breakthrough migraines.

One example of an obscure trigger turned out to be scallops and prawns. When fresh, I could consume small amounts without issue; however, frozen or marinated versions had a more detrimental effect. Prior to discovering this, I was becoming confident in my understanding of which foods and drinks to avoid, but I still could not figure out what was causing my early morning headaches and midmorning breakthrough migraines. Revisiting my migraine diary, I noticed a pattern: on three different occasions, I had consumed a pre-frozen scallop. Because I'm a glutton for punishment, I decided to confirm my findings by preparing another portion of those scallops. The tell-tale signs reappeared early the next morning, confirming the link between scallops and my migraine episodes. I also noticed the same issue with prawns.

Another important observation in my diary was an increased susceptibility to triggers during my hormonal cycle. While I could consume small amounts of certain trigger foods without consequences earlier in the month, I noticed that a few days before my period, I became more sensitive to these foods, and migraines would be more severe and longer lasting.

Ultimately, the migraine diary became an invaluable tool in my journey towards understanding and managing my migraines. What began as a simple record of symptoms evolved into a profound guide, uncovering patterns that were previously hidden. By meticulously tracking triggers, whether food related, hormonal or stress induced, I gained significant insights into the complex nature of my migraines.

As I reflect on my journey, I'm excited and proud to have finally kicked that migraine for good.

This journey has been long and challenging, but it represents a significant personal victory for me.

While I still need to be mindful of my triggers, I can now enjoy foods I once couldn't. Occasionally, if I push those limits, I might wake up with a mild headache, but it's nothing compared to the debilitating pain I once endured. Instead, they are gentle reminders of my journey. Today, I feel empowered, more connected with my body, my wellbeing and more in control of my future.

CHAPTER 1

What Doctors Don't Tell You

1.1 Why Conventional Migraine Medication is Ineffective

Conventional migraine medications have shown numerous shortcomings, with many migraine sufferers experiencing little or no relief. Poor outcomes can lead to potential overreliance of pain medication, associated with a growing number of reported cases, raising alarms about the substantial adverse effects linked to commonly used migraine drugs.

Adverse effects, often called side effects, are unintended and undesirable symptoms of a drug. They can occur with both synthetic and natural drugs, but synthetic drugs, due to their complexity and the potential for off-target effects, may exhibit a wider range of adverse effects.

Consequently, there is a pressing need to explore therapeutic alternatives that offer effective relief with fewer potential adverse side effects. By adopting a holistic approach, healthcare providers can tailor treatments to the unique needs and circumstances of each patient. This can help reduce the reliance on medications and greatly improve treatment outcomes. Additionally, promoting awareness among both healthcare professionals and the general public about the risks associated with overusing triptans and nonsteroidal anti-inflammatory Drugs (NSAIDs) is crucial.

In this chapter, I will provide you with some eye-opening information on current migraine medication, including the often-overlooked risk of adverse effects from these drugs that nobody tells you about.

Additionally, I will discuss medication overuse, which can lead to rebound headaches (migraine), and provide important information on drug tolerance, when the effectiveness of the medication decreases with continued use.

But firstly, I will provide some important insights into the heterogeneous condition of migraines and why pharmaceutical treatments are not effective.

1.2 The Heterogeneous Condition of Migraines

With a background in medicine, and years of experience working with migraine patients, I have come to the conclusion that migraines are perhaps the most convoluted and complex condition of the human body. This is precisely why there is still no efficient treatment, let alone a cure.

The first factor contributing to the limitations of migraine medication is the heterogenous nature of migraines. Migraines are diverse and varied in nature and no single treatment approach will provide a satisfactory outcome. They are highly individual, much like a fingerprint, with sufferers presenting different characteristics, including a wide range of symptoms that can occur in different combinations, with varying degrees of severity and frequency.

Triggers can also vary greatly from person to person and are influenced by the environment, lifestyle, diet, and the individual's stress profile. Additionally, different people will respond to different treatments for migraines. All these factors contribute to the heterogeneous nature of migraines, making it difficult to develop a one-size-fits-all approach to manage their condition. Furthermore, the personalised nature of migraines and the patient's unique characteristics not only leads to the ineffectiveness of drugs and the need for a combination of medications to improve efficacy, but also makes selecting the right medication a trial-and-error process.

1.3 Synthetically Based Drugs with Selective Targeting Capacity

There are several limitations of contemporary migraine medications, one of which is their synthetic makeup, which can result in a higher incidence of adverse effects since the body may not recognise the chemical composition as readily as medications derived from natural sources.

Furthermore, pharmaceuticals are generally developed as 'selective targeting' drugs. For example, migraine medications like triptans and CGRP inhibitors are designed for this purpose.

Selective targeting drugs are more potent and more particular in targeting a specific molecule or pathway with the intention of achieving a specific therapeutic effect.

The downside of selective targeting drugs is the increased risk of adverse effects because the target molecule or pathway may have multiple functions in the body, and the drug may interfere with these functions, leading to unintended adverse effects—a notable characteristic of synthetic drugs.

Additionally, the targeting of a specific pathway can lead to compensatory changes in other pathways due to the loss of function in the target pathway, which can further increase the risk of adverse effects.

The adverse effect of selective targeting of neurotransmitters and their receptors in migraine medication serves as a quintessential example of precision-based treatment, illustrating how drugs can interfere with other pathways beyond their primary targets.

In contrast to synthetic medications, natural plant-derived active compounds tend to be more complex and multifaceted. They generally have a broader range of active compounds that can interact with multiple receptors and enzymes. As a result, they often have a gentle impact on the body and therefore fewer side effects. Nevertheless, it is important to keep in mind that despite being derived from natural sources, natural medicines can also have potent effects and should always be used with caution and under the guidance of a health professional.

1.4 Medication Overuse

An additional and significant limitation is medication overuse. A condition in which individuals use medication excessively, often leading to negative effects or worsening of their condition. This term is commonly used in the context of headaches, where overuse of pain medications can result in more frequent or severe headaches. In the medical community, this is termed medication overuse headache (MOH) and is also known as a 'rebound headache' or 'analgesic headache'.[2]

MOH typically develops in individuals who use headache medications more than two to three times per week. This overuse of migraine medication initiates a cycle of increasing headache and migraine frequency, leading to more medication consumption, ultimately exacerbating headache and migraine pain.

MOH is difficult to treat and often requires a reduction or elimination of the offending medication, which is a serious dilemma when you suffer from severe migraine episodes. In contrast, complementary medicine is designed to restore health and eliminate the underlying causes of the migraine condition. An example of this would include avoiding triggers, adapting the nervous system to reduce hypersensitivities, and breaking the inflammatory and stress cycle to restore brain plasticity.

1.5 Drug Tolerance

Lastly, another limitation is the occurrence of drug tolerance, where the effectiveness of the medication decreases with continued use. This phenomenon, known as compensatory adaptation or compensatory response, occurs as the body tries to maintain homeostasis in response to the initial intervention. The implications of this are that firstly, it can reduce the effectiveness of the treatment over time as the body adapts to counteract the effects of the drug. This can result in the need for higher doses or alternative treatments to achieve the desired effect.

Secondly, compensatory changes in other pathways can lead to unintended adverse effects. An example with triptan medication is chest symptoms, including tightness, pressure, or pain in the chest or throat. The exact mechanism behind chest symptoms as an adverse effect of triptans is not fully understood. However, it is believed that the vasoconstrictive effect of triptans may also affect blood vessels in other parts of the body, including the coronary arteries that supply the heart. This could potentially lead to chest symptoms such as tightness, pressure or pain. It is important to seek medical attention if you experience these symptoms while taking triptans.

Drug tolerance is a common issue with long-term pain management drugs, particularly those used for migraines. Ultimately, the limited availability of effective pharmaceutical migraine medication, coupled with frequent adverse effects, makes it a poorly tolerated treatment option.

1.6 The Dark Side of Migraine Medication

At this point, I have provided some insight into why conventional medicine struggles to effectively treat migraines. In this section, I will shed some light on the true nature of several commonly used migraine medications, including triptans, ditans, ergotamine, and calcitonin gene-related peptide inhibitors (CGRP), and reveal the lesser-known, darker aspects of these medications that are typically not discussed by your practitioner or pharmacist.

Based on my research and clinical experience with migraine patients, I have found that these drugs often fail to yield the desired results and can lead to unintended adverse effects that outweigh any potential benefits.

In the current conventional approach to migraine treatment, medications are classified into two categories: acute and chronic. These medications are often used in combination therapy, which involves utilising two distinct medications with the goal of achieving a common therapeutic outcome. Using two drugs is not uncommon due to the inadequacy of single therapy in addressing the complex nature of migraines. Hence, utilising two different medications that target different aspects of the migraine process may result in improved outcomes. For instance, a combination of a triptan and a non-steroidal anti-inflammatory drug can be utilised to enhance relief from both headache pain and associated symptoms, such as nausea and vomiting.

The acute category of medication includes triptans, ditans, ergotamine, opioids and non-steroidal anti-inflammatory medication, used for symptomatic relief and only taken when a migraine is imminent. One of the challenges with acute medication administration is that it is frequently delayed, resulting in poor efficacy. The elusive and unpredictable nature of migraines can make it difficult to identify premonitory symptoms, and if not recognised in a timely manner, the window of opportunity for effective treatment may be missed, reducing the chances of a successful outcome. Furthermore, any oral migraine medication that requires absorption through the stomach is generally ineffective if delayed, as the stomach of individuals experiencing migraines may shut down and thus prevent absorption of the medication.

Having discussed short-term migraine medications, it's also important to understand long-term migraine medication, which is used for individuals with frequent or severe migraines. This type of medication is often referred to as 'preventative' migraine medication. Typical long-term medications include beta blockers, calcium channel blockers, antiepileptics, antidepressants, and Botox. While these medications were originally developed for other conditions, they have been found to provide some relief for severe and chronic migraine cases. They are considered effective if they reduce migraine frequency or severity by at least 50%.[3] Similar results appear in a large-meta-analysis (50,000 participants), which reported the proportion of patients achieved less than a 50% reduction in headache frequency.[4] Admittedly, not a great result.

Due to these drugs' ineffectivenesss, they are often combined with an acute, symptomatic relief medication as an adjunct when a migraine is imminent. Although patients have some welcome reprieve from their torment, these drugs augment a poor response and are generally not well tolerated due to their adverse effects. Let's explore some of these commonly used drugs more closely to uncover their true nature.

1.7 Triptans

Triptans are synthetic drugs that target three specific serotonin receptors, known as 5-HT-1B/1D/1F. These receptors have different functions in the body. The 5-HT1B receptors are located on cranial blood vessels and cause constrict, reducing blood flow. The 5-HT1D receptors are mainly found in trigeminal nerve fibres and inhibit the release of CGRP, a vasodilatory neuropeptide involved in migraine pain. Finally, the 5-HT1F receptors inhibit the production of pain signals.[5,6]

It's important to note that triptans can act in two ways: they can either activate receptor activity (agonistic) or inhibit it (antagonistic). This means they can selectively target certain receptors to achieve specific effects. Some triptans have shown functional selectivity for certain receptors, which allows them to be more effective in treating migraines.

Although triptans can target three primary serotonin receptors, their effectiveness varies widely. Approximately 45% of triptan users do not experience relief, and many also report adverse effects.[7] Common adverse effects include dizziness, drowsiness, fatigue, dry mouth, nausea, muscle weakness, and flushing. Some users can experience severe symptoms such as breathing difficulties, racing heart, severe neck, jaw, chest and shoulder pain, tingling and numbness in legs and arms, and panic attacks.[8]

The vasoconstrictive effects of the 5-HT1B receptors has been linked to stroke and heart attack and are not recommended for people with cardiovascular issues. Triptans are not used as a preventative medicine, and like anti-inflammatories and ergotamine, they need to be taken acutely and timely for a favourable result.

1.8 Ditans

Ditans are a newer class of triptans that target the 5-HT1F receptor, inhibiting the release of inflammatory compounds, specifically substance P, CGRP and glutamate. This helps reduce pain and vasodilation associated with migraines. Unlike older triptans, ditans do not cause vasoconstriction, making them a better option for migraine patients with cardiovascular disorders.

Nevertheless, it is imperative to acknowledge that the scope of 5-HT1F receptor function extends beyond merely modulating pain. These receptors play a crucial role in regulating mood, emotion and sleep regulation. Consequently, the drug will impact these physiological processes, leading to potential side effects.

Lasmiditan, which was approved in 2019, is the first and only ditan on the market and remains a relatively novel pharmaceutical agent. Its recent introduction provides a limited understanding of the potential adverse effects. My best option was to do a search on the FDA Adverse Event Reporting System (FAERS). This is a system used by healthcare providers and patients who can report adverse effects of prescribed drugs. Keeping in mind though that this is a voluntary reporting system, and the figures indicating the number of adverse events is only what has been reported, this is not a true reflection of all medication users.

The FAERS reported summary of adverse events for Lasmiditan, encompassed a total of 798 patients between 2020 and 2022. Of these reports, 68 were considered serious cases, including 11 deaths.[9] The most common adverse effects reported were dizziness 23.5 %, feeling abnormal 13.5%, drowsiness 12%, drug ineffectiveness 10.5%, migraine 4%, and headache 3%. Users also complained of nausea, vomiting, anxiety, and changes in blood pressure and heart rate.[9] This constitutes a substantial number of serious adverse outcomes, particularly given the limited sample size and brief time frame considered. These results emphasise the importance of the severity of negative events linked to Lasmiditan.

The FDA Adverse Event Reporting System (FAERS) is a system dedicated to tracking and monitoring adverse events specifically related to drug use. This includes a range of unexpected outcomes individuals may experience when taking a particular drug, such as drug interactions, side effects and other unintended reactions.

1.9 Ergotamine

Ergotamine is the only non-synthetic migraine medication. It is noteworthy that ergotamine was the first medication to be introduced for the treatment of migraines and remains one of the most reliable and effective options, with minimal adverse effects when used correctly.

Additionally, dihydroergotamine, a semisynthetic derivative of ergot is also available. This modified molecule structure might offer longer-lasting effects and be less potent in causing vasoconstriction.[10]

Before I discuss the benefits of Ergotamine as a treatment for migraines, it is imperative to shed some light on the historical significance of this substance.

In 1925, a Swiss physician by the name of Dr Ernst Maier was the first to use Ergotamine on his patients for the acute treatment of migraines, and reported significant improvements in their symptoms.[11] This marked the beginning of Ergotamine use and established it as one of the first effective treatments for this condition.

In 1938, Graham and Wolff demonstrated that Ergotamine not only reduced migraine pain, but also led to the constriction of the dilated temporal artery.[12] However, like most natural-based medicines, the discovery of Ergotamine was through trial and error. The natural compound is derived from the highly toxic fungi Claviceps purpurea, found growing on cultivated grains like rye, wheat and barley. The historical documentation of ergot poisoning was recorded as far back as 600 BC by the Assyrians, but the peak of recorded incidences of ergotism was during the Middle Ages when grains like rye became a staple food. The consumption of ergot contaminated rye made into bread flour had a devastating death toll on many communities.

With the advancement in chemistry and pharmacology, it became evident that ergot alkaloids, although highly toxic, have a therapeutic potential in very small doses, which eventually led to the first migraine medication in the second half of the 19th century.[13]

The therapeutic concentrations of Ergotamine and Dihydroergotamine act as an agonist on the serotonin receptors and the monoamine receptors dopamine, epinephrine and norepinephrine.[14] The most potent activity is on the serotonin receptors 5HT1B and 5HT1D.[15] The activation of these receptors induces constriction of intracranial and extracerebral blood vessels, inhibits trigeminal neurotransmission and terminates neurogenic inflammation and pain. [12][15] The best choice for the administration of Ergotamine are suppositories (Ergotamine 2 mg with caffeine 100 mg). These are administered rectally and are less likely to cause nausea and vomiting compared to the oral alternative. Other options are nasal spray (Dihydroergotamine Mesylate 2 mg) and sublingual tablets (Ergotamine tartrate 2 mg), but nausea and vomiting are still common, with a plausibility that some of the sublingual medicine ends up in the gastric system.

From a clinical experience, I have found that the common dosage of 2 mg of Ergotamine (suppository) is mostly excessive and therefore more likely to present with unwanted side effects such as nausea and vomiting, muscle pain and neuralgia type symptoms.

It is ideal to experiment with smaller dozes by reducing the size of the tablet or suppository and see what amount has the best outcome for you personally. Some patients can have a satisfactory result with a third or even a quarter suppository. Again, the timing of administration is important for an optimal outcome. Relief of symptoms should occur around 20-30 minutes if taken with the first premonitions of an imminent migraine.

In many countries, the availability of Ergotamine and Dihydroergotamine medicine is becoming more difficult as the pharmaceutical trend for migraine medicine is pushing more cost-effective drugs like triptans and CGRPs. In Australia, Ergotamine has been taken off the shelves and is not recommended by general practitioners unless the patient specifically asks for a prescription prepared by a compounding pharmacist.

1.10 CGRP Inhibitor

The calcitonin gene-related peptide inhibitors (CGRPs) are the latest novel preventative medication for migraines that has emerged on the market in recent years. CGRP inhibitors come in two types. The first on the market at the end of 2019 where gepants, a receptor antagonist that blocks the CGRP receptors to stop inflammation and vasodilation. This is an oral medication and is mostly used for acute treatment or it is combined with a triptan or anti-inflammatory.

In 2020, the first monoclonal antibody CGRP inhibitor was released, which is a synthetic protein that attaches to the surface of the CGRP messenger or the receptor and alters its shape to make it unrecognisable. It also provides the same therapeutic outcome as gepants. Due to the large molecular structure of this drug, the application needs to be subcutaneous injections or intravenous infusion on a monthly or quarterly basis.

There has been significant hype surrounding CGRP inhibitors since their introduction to the market, but the quality and efficacy of this drug is greatly exaggerated when considering user reviews. Comparative analysis suggests that the positive effects of CGRP inhibitors may be relatively weaker than other migraine medications. For instance, according to a medicine review, the therapeutic gain of CGRP inhibitors is less than 10% compared to placebo. In contrast, the therapeutic gain for triptans falls between 16-21%[16] which, while better, is not particularly impressive either.

The FAERS database results for the injectable CGRP monoclonal antibodies is not promising either. According to Robbins MD (2020), the reporting system for the end of 2019 lists 24,643 adverse events linked to three brands of CGRP monoclonal antibodies—erenumab, fremanezumab, and galcanezumab. Among these, there were 3,520 life-threatening events and 126 deaths.[16]

These are striking figures, especially considering this medicine has been on the market for just under two years. Such numbers are certainly not acceptable. While there is a place for serious drugs where the potential benefits outweigh the risks, migraines should by no means fall into this category.

To put this into perspective, when I compared these results with Ergotamine tartrate in the reporting system, I found that in the same time frame, there were a total of 209 reported adverse events spanning from 1969 to 2022, with 186 serious events and six deaths.[17] It is important to note that this Ergotamine event report spans over 54 years, in stark contrast to the two-year timeframe for CGRP monoclonal antibodies.

Due to the limited market exposure, the long-term risks of CGRP inhibitors remain unknown, and it may take more than a decade before we can observe any serious outcomes.

A good example of a long-term migraine medication is Methysergide, which was discontinued at the end of 2013. methysergide was sold under the brand names Sansert and Deseril, and it was taken daily as a preventative medicine. The withdrawal of the drug is due to retroperitoneal and pulmonary fibrosis. The FAERS database results included a total of 761 cases during 1969-2022. Of these, 104 patients were diagnosed with retroperitoneal fibrosis and 32 with pulmonary fibrosis. There were also 21 deaths.[18]

The information on adverse effects of CGRP inhibitors is available, but practitioners often do not share this information with patients, which can hinder the patient's ability to make an informed choice. Clinical studies that evaluate the drug's efficacy and safety are currently all short term and do not reveal its long-term adverse effects. However, as the drug becomes more commonly used, migraine clinics and patients share treatment outcomes and experiences on platforms such as drugs.com and webmd.com. Such anecdotal information can offer valuable insights for individuals seeking to make well-informed decisions about their treatment options.

To have a better understanding on the most frequent adverse effects, I did another search on the FAERS database with the inclusion of a combination of both CGRP gepants and monoclonal antibodies. The result included 1,696 patients and the most frequent adverse effects included drug ineffectiveness 14%, migraine 13%, nausea 12%, constipation 11%, fatigue 7%, hair loss 2%, digestive issues like constipation, reflux, gastritis 2-4%, weight gain, changes in blood pressure and heart rate,[19] and so the list goes on.

It is not surprising that inhibiting this receptor can result in unintended consequences. From an evolutionary standpoint, CGRP has evolved to serve a critical regulatory function in the immune and cardiovascular system, reducing the risk of stroke and heart attack, aiding in wound healing, and supporting optimal gastric function.[20] Its potent vasodilatory effect is integral in maintaining and regulating blood pressure and oxygen-carrying capacity.[20]

1.11 Botox

OnabotulinumtoxinA, commonly known as Botox, is a versatile medication utilised for various conditions, including migraines. Its mechanism of action involves blocking the release of certain neurotransmitters that are involved in pain signals, which can help to reduce the frequency and severity of migraines.

Botox is usually given as a series of injections into the muscle of the head, neck and shoulders. The injections are typically given every 12 weeks and the exact number of injections required can vary based on the individual's needs. Some people may require more frequent injections, while others may be able to extend the time between treatments. The medication takes several days to start working, so relief from migraines may not be immediate.

Adverse effects of Botox can include injection site pain, neck pain, muscle weakness, eye disorders, and skin allergy reactions. It can also cause muscle weakness, double vision or difficulty in speaking. In rare cases, the spread of the toxin beyond the injection site can cause serious and potentially life-threatening problems such as difficulty breathing or swallowing, respiratory failure or cardiac arrest.[21]

Brain Bites and Guided Strategies

1. As you have learned so far, conventional medicine has its limitations in terms of adverse effects, should not be recommended for long-term use, and more often than not has inadequate symptom relief.

Nevertheless, it can improve the quality of life in the short term and serve as a useful bridging tool as you transition to a complementary treatment plan. Combining both approaches can achieve a better short-term outcome and maintain your quality of life.

I would also encourage that you work with your complementary healthcare provider for guidance and address any questions you may have during this transition.

CHAPTER 2

Getting to Know Your Personal Triggers and Premonition Symptoms

2.1 The Migraine Brain

During my research, I came across a fascinating article of a peculiar condition that some migraine sufferers experience called Alice in Wonderland Syndrome (AIWS). Reading this article a sudden realisation hit me, it was a perfect description of something I had unknowingly experienced as a child. I vividly remember how my arms or body would swell, almost like the Michelin Man. It was a peculiar sensation, yet oddly pleasant, and it only happened at night just before I fell asleep.

This syndrome is a rare and intriguing neurological phenomenon of perceptual alterations of one's body. Individuals may perceive their limbs or even their entire body as expanding like an inflated balloon. It often comes with a range of perceptual anomalies, creating a dreamlike or hallucinatory quality to the experience. The phenomenon is named after Lewis Carroll's famous novel, *Alice's Adventures in Wonderland*, where the principal character, Alice, encounters a world filled with bizarre and unpredictable changes in size and perspective. While the exact causes of AIWS are still not fully understood, researchers have observed that it often associated with migraines, epilepsy or viral brain infections.[22] In particular, the 'migraine brain' shows unique differences from a non-migraine brain, especially in how it processes sensory information, often with an intense sensitivity that can make experiences more vivid, disorienting or overwhelming.

The migraine condition is a complex neurological process characterised by severe symptoms, including debilitating headaches, nausea, vomiting, and fatigue. While not all migraines are severe, they can be extremely debilitating for some individuals, significantly impacting their quality of life during an attack. However, identifying the myriad of factors that can trigger migraines is formidable, contributing to the challenge of effectively treating the condition and often resulting in poor treatment outcomes.

These challenges arise because migraines originate from the nervous and endocrine systems, and certain sensory inputs, known as triggers, lead the brain to process this sensory information differently.

There is a myriad of triggers, ranging from those that can be explained, like food sensitivities, mental stressors and hormonal changes, towards more obscure and challenging triggers, such as atmospheric variations and lunar cycles, which influence biological conditions. These triggers, while not fully understood by science, can have a significant impact on some individuals.

Specific traits that may influence the sensitivity of the migraine brain are genetic variations in the way enzymes and receptors function on a cellular level. These variations can influence many metabolic pathways and how certain stimuli are processed in the brain. However, the most remarkable aspect of a migraine brain is its heightened susceptibility to perceived stressors, with stress being one of the foremost triggers for migraines.

Through my clinical experience, I have noticed that migraineurs have a highly refined nervous system, which also brings with it a heightened sense of smell, taste and hearing. This heightened sensitivity of the sensory organs makes one more attuned to the surrounding environment. On the flip side, this finely tuned system is also more vulnerable to perceived stress. During a migraine episode, these exceptionally heightened senses, particularly to sound and light, can feel as debilitating as kryptonite is to Superman.

Whether physical or emotional, these sensitivities will bring various vulnerabilities for migraine sufferers, the most common of which is headaches. For many, stressors can trigger tension headaches, which can often progress to a migraine episode.

A tension headache is a type of headache that often results from a combination of physical and mental stressors. These headaches involve the neuroendocrine system, which includes the release of hormones and neurotransmitters in response to the sympathetic nervous system, also known as the stress response.

One primary factor contributing to tension headaches is the exertion of muscles in the upper body, particularly in the shoulders and neck. This can be caused by various factors, including mental and emotional stress, as well as poor posture.

Poor posture has become increasingly prevalent in modern society, largely due to the use of electronic gadgets. Office workers and students, often adopt postures that are not ergonomic, leading to muscle strain and tension headaches. Additionally, repetitive movements and insufficient breaks from such static positions can also contribute to poor posture and tension headaches.

Other common triggers for tension headaches include hunger or fasting, overexertion from physical activity, and eye strain.

Like poor posture, eye strain is a common trigger for tension headaches, aggravated by poor lighting, extended focus on electronic screens, or issues with focus. If you frequently experience tension headaches and have symptoms like irritated or burning dry eyes, or pressure behind the eyes, you might have a condition called visually induced 'trigeminal dysphoria', which is a visual misalignment between the two eyes. This condition has become more prevalent with the widespread use of digital devices. If you think you suffer from eye strain and it may contribute as a trigger to your headaches or migraine, I recommend you make an appointment with your optometrist for an assessment. You can also find helpful exercises tips at the end of this section under 'Brain Bites and Guided Strategies'.

Keep in mind that you will have your own unique symptoms and triggers for tension-type headaches, which only you can identify. Some symptoms may be bold and obvious, while others will be elusive, and it will take some time to recognise these. Therefore, it is important to note everything in your symptom diary so that you can identify emerging patterns. The earlier you can intervene in your tension headache, the more successful you will be in reducing the frequency of your migraine episodes.

Tension headaches typically develop slowly, with symptoms appearing up to eight hours before the headache itself. Some of these symptoms may resemble those of a migraine. They often start subtly, such as with aching in the back, shoulders and neck, or a vague irritation in the eyes.

As these symptoms progress, you might unconsciously rub your neck or shoulders, stretch your lower back, or feel affected by electronic screens or room lighting. At this stage, you might even feel slightly irritated or short-tempered with your current task. Ignoring these early, subtle symptoms without taking a break can lead to a full-blown tension headache.

It's wise to become familiar with the symptom pattern of your tension headaches and start preventive measures early.

A tension headache is often described as a dull, aching pain, that feels like a tight band around the head. Some may liken it to a vice-like grip, feeling pressure or tightness on the forehead or back of the head, or experiencing a deep-seated pressure. Unlike migraine headaches, tension headaches are not typically affected by lying down or physical activity.

As a tension headache progresses, some tell-tale migraine symptoms may emerge. Pain may become more localised, affecting areas such as the base of the skull, forehead, temples, upper and lower jaw, and behind the eyes. At this stage, natural remedies often prove insufficient to halt the inflammatory process, necessitating the use of typical migraine medication. With limited options at this point, the priority shifts to halting the inflammatory process and considering your overall well-being.

To manage tension headaches and halt the inflammatory process, a suitable non-steroidal anti-inflammatory drug (NSAID) can be effective. It's possible that you already have a preferred medication that works for you.

Fine-tuning your skill in identifying the type of headache will be challenging and not without its setbacks, but with dedicated practice it will eventually become easier to judge. Regularly noting this information in your migraine diary will help you to identify your personal trigger patterns over time.

Differentiating between migraine headaches and other types of headaches can be challenging since migraine sufferers are generally susceptible to headaches. Even for experienced migraineurs, it can be a lottery whether their current headache symptoms will evolve into a migraine. In this situation, the question arises as to whether to take migraine medication or not. The reluctance to take medication in the belief that it is just a mild headache often results in delayed and ineffective treatment. Delayed medication can also occur at night during sleep. Migraines have an affinity to develop in the middle of the night and consequently wake you due to the discomfort of headache pain. If you wake too late or ignore the head pain in your slumber, any oral medication at this stage is often ineffective, as digestion has ceased, and the drug is not able to be absorbed.

The pain of a migraine headache can vary from an unmistakable throbbing pain, usually concentrated on one side of the head, to a heavy, dull pain deep in the skull. Pain is the hallmark symptom of a migraine headache, marking the peak of the migraine process, where localised areas of dilated and constricted blood vessels in specific brain regions are at their most vulnerable. A migraine headache is exacerbated by physical activity and lying down, which increases blood pressure and pulsation on the vulnerable blood vessels.

The pain may shift and gradually intensify, varying from person to person. The accompanying symptoms are also uniquely individual and can include visual aura, nausea, vomiting, diarrhoea, fatigue, or temporary loss of vision and weakness on one side of the body. These symptoms can also extend to certain sensitivities especially light, sound and odours, and can intensify the throbbing head pain.

It's important to note that not all types of migraine are characterised by a headache. Silent migraines, digestive migraines and vestibular migraines may or may not be associated with headache pain. These types are typically characterised by their own unique symptoms, including fatigue, vertigo or dizziness, and nausea and vomiting.

Migraine is a complex condition, and each person's experience is unique, much like a fingerprint. Identifying the factors that trigger migraines can be intricate and challenging due to the complex interactions between metabolic pathways, epigenetics, environment, and lifestyle factors. The best way to unravel this complexity is through anecdotal evidence. In other words, understanding the individuality of migraines and their impact on patients' lives is often better achieved through individual cases rather than relying solely on rigorous scientific research or clinical trials. As a clinician, I rely on my patients' personal experiences and accounts, as well as my own clinical expertise, to understand and manage their migraines effectively.

The migraine process, from trigger to headache, involves intricate biochemical events that engage the endocrine, immune and neurovascular systems. A communications process facilitated by miniscule chemical messengers including enzymes, hormones and neurotransmitters. Fundamentally, these physiological communication networks form the foundation in regulating the body's equilibrium, an innate process known as homeostasis. These networks are responsible for things like maintaining blood pressure, body temperature, electrolyte and pH balance. However, during a migraine episode, these communication pathways react more intensely, leading to a cascade of events that disrupts normal homeostasis.

Migraines are no exception; numerous pathological factors contribute to the disruption of the equilibrium. Common factors such as infections, allergies, food intolerances, nutrient deficiencies, digestive issues, stress, and chronic disease, to name a few. When we feel unwell, the body's organised frenzy of neuroendocrine and immune responses produces symptoms that we are only too familiar with, including aches and pain, fatigue, fever, nausea, diarrhoea, and just feeling poorly.

A notable example in migraine pathology is the inordinate vasomotor activity observed in cerebral blood vessels. In other words, there is a disproportionate impact on blood vessels, either constricting or dilating. The excessive vasoconstriction and consequent vasodilation is unique to the migraine process and correlates in the regions where pain is present. The typical intensely and distinctive throbbing pain relates to the pulsatile blood flow and typically worsens with physical activity and lying down. Although the primary and most obvious migraine pathology is expressed in the brain during the headache phase, the presentation of symptomatic events occurs much earlier and are highly individual with every migraineur. I will discuss this in more detail in the forthcoming chapters about the four phases of a migraine.

The term 'migraine attack' is commonly used in literature, and also seems to be the primary focus for researchers in the pathology of migraines. This term seems to denote an instant ambush of a migraine headache, which is ambiguous as migraines do not appear suddenly but evolve over time. The process of an evolving migraine is not obvious to the untrained eye, making it difficult to perceive or recognise certain traits within this process. However, the term 'attack' conveys the intense and often debilitating nature of the throbbing headache pain experienced during a migraine. Another term you will frequently encounter in this book is 'migraine episode.

This term encompasses the entire pathophysiological progression of a migraine, which unfolds in four distinct phases: the trigger phase, the premonition phase, the headache phase, and recovery phase.

Brain Bites and Guided Strategies

- The migraine brain is characterised by heightened sensory perceptions that are highly sensitive to the external environment and internal stressors.

- Underlying imbalances such as inflammation, oxidative stress, nutritional deficiencies, and metabolic dysfunction may contribute to this heightened sensitivity

- Tension headaches are common in migraineurs and result from a combination of mental stressors and physiological stressors such as poor posture, hunger, overexertion, and eye strain.

- Recognising the early symptoms of tension headaches can help prevent them from progressing into full-blown migraines.

- Helpful exercises and advice for eye care, such as managing eye strain and trigeminal dysphoria, are available in The Therapy Kit (Chapter 5, Section 5.6).

2.2 Four Phases of a Migraine Episode

The migraine process is a sequence of pathophysiological events, which can be divided into four distinct phases. The first phase, the trigger phase, begins when a specific factor initiates a migraine attack. Next comes the premonition phase, which is characterised by subtle and imperceptible symptoms that signal the onset of the headache phase. The headache phase is the main event of the attack and involves intense pain and other symptoms. The postdrome or recovery phase is the end of the migraine episode and is characterised by residual symptoms and general fatigue. Unlike the headache phase, the trigger phase and premonition phases are notoriously difficult to identify and have a development phase of between 2- 48 hours before it reaches the headache phase.

The nature of migraines is typically random and unpredictable. They have a tendency to sneak up on you and once the headache pain commences, the opportunity for any intervention is mostly too late. I often use the metaphor of a dormant volcano to describe migraines. Without the right tools to identify the subtle warning signs, such as the deep rumblings in the earth, it's impossible to predict when the volcano will erupt. Similarly, the elusive rumblings of a migraine can occur hours or even days before a full-blown attack, making it difficult to prepare and manage the symptoms. By learning to recognise these early warning signs, you have the ability to take steps to prevent or minimise the impact of a migraine.

In this chapter, I will provide a comprehensive overview of the four phases, including a detailed explanation of how they develop. I will also equip you with the knowledge to recognise the first signs and symptoms and offer strategies to intervene and halt the process using appropriate tools.

2.3 The Trigger Phase

The trigger phase is the first stage in the migraine process. It is the silent phase during which physiological changes are set in motion—and we are oblivious to its occurrence. Triggers comprise a broad and diverse group of chemical substances which are present in our diet and the environment we live in, some of which are produced within our body. The incubation period for a trigger to the progressive stage of a migraine attack can range from 2-48 hours, depending on the migraineur's state of susceptibility to triggers and sensitivity to the internal pathological process. The susceptibility and sensitivity in a migraine episode significantly influences both the frequency and severity of migraines. Understanding these two factors is crucial for developing effective treatment strategies.

Susceptibility to migraines is strongly influenced by the body's response to a variety of triggers. Factors like nutrient deficiencies, frequent infections, digestive issues, autoimmune conditions, and glucose dysregulation can increase vulnerability as they contribute to a state of heightened inflammation and oxidative stress. While a typically highly sensitive nervous system is the foundation for the migraine sufferer, these predisposing factors further heighten the neurological sensitivity and susceptibility to triggers. Neurological sensitivity varies significantly among individuals, with chronic migraine sufferers being the most susceptible to triggers, even with minimal exposure.

Identifying your triggers marks a significant victory in the battle against migraines. However, the crux of the matter lies in pinpointing your unique personal triggers, which constitutes the primary challenge in this journey. While the triggers provided by your physician or discovered online offer a skeletal framework, they merely represent a fraction of the myriad of potential triggers that can induce a migraine.

To master your personal triggers, you will find that the trigger phase is the most significant stage in the strategies to conquer your migraine. I will guide you through all the known triggers that can instigate a migraine episode and provide you with the tools to help recognise and avoid your own personal migraine triggers. Firstly, we need to understand what a trigger is and its involvement in initiating the very first immune response. It is important to note that triggers are highly distinctive for each person and can be devilishly elusive and unpredictable. Importantly, the only way to get to know your personal triggers is through personal experience.

In my early twenties, I discovered that fortified wine, particularly sherry, triggered my migraines. At that time, I had no idea that alcoholic beverages could cause migraines, however, the link with sherry was unmistakable. Within a couple of hours, I would inevitably experience a severe migraine. Unfortunately, it took three occasions at my lovely neighbour's home bar, where I was served sherry in crystal glasses, before I made the connection.

At that time, I knew very little about my migraines. Now, I understand the implications of sherry's long fermentation process, which leads to a substantial accumulation of amines, high levels of acetaldehyde, and not to mention a high alcohol content of 15 to 22%—a perfect cocktail for the mother of all migraines.

Most migraine triggers are not as obvious as my experience with sherry. Triggers can stem from a broad variety of diverse sources, can interact with other triggers, and the varying degrees of an individual's sensitivity can make identifying triggers extremely challenging.

2.4 Identifying your Triggers: Factors that Influence a Migraine Episode

If you suffer from migraines that are either frequent or severe or have a long duration, your body is more reactive to certain triggers, and it is an indication of increased tissue sensitivity. This increased sensitivity stems from an imbalance in the neuroendocrine and immune system that renders a rapid and severe inflammatory response every time there is a trigger encounter.

There are several factors contributing to an increased sensitivity. Firstly, being a stress head will make you more susceptible to any external and especially *internal* triggers, as stress will always be the driving force. Any current underlying condition or disease will result an increased susceptibility as the body is already dealing with inflammation and the immune system is ready and primed. Typical conditions which intensify immune response can include food intolerances, allergies, digestive problems including an imbalance of the gut microbiome (dysbiosis), and blood sugar dysregulation.

Increased sensitivity is also influenced by the extent of exposure to a trigger. This heightened exposure to triggers and resulting migraines leads to a change in brain plasticity, an adaptive mechanism that increases responsiveness and sensitivity to subsequent triggers. If you would like to learn more about how brain plasticity is involved with migraines, please refer to Section 4.4 in Chapter 4.

Another frequent trigger I have observed in clients is poor posture, which can lead to recurrent symptoms of back, shoulder or neck pain. Poor posture is a common issue among office workers, often stemming from inadequate ergonomics at computer workstations. Susceptibility to migraines increases with poor posture, especially when symptoms are ignored in favour of finishing tasks without taking breaks. Conversely, while a lack of physical activity and poor muscle integrity can contribute to migraines, excessive physical activity involving the shoulder complex, such as hard physical work or intense weightlifting in the gym, can also initiate a neurological process that may trigger migraines.

Any strenuous activity that causes physical exertion can act as a trigger. Both physical and mental stressors activate the same neurological pathways, allowing body tissues to adapt. While this adaptation process is beneficial in moderation, excessive or prolonged stress can overwhelm the body's coping mechanisms and result in negative health effects.[23]

If you're susceptible to migraines triggered through physical exertion, it's important to strike a balance in your physical activity levels. This approach promotes overall wellbeing and helps minimise the risk of migraine triggers.

Migraines can also be triggered by excessive sweating, often due to an electrolyte imbalance, particularly deficiencies in sodium and magnesium. Personally, as an avid hiker, I used to experience migraines at the end of a strenuous long walk, especially on hot days. Adding a little extra salt to my diet made a significant difference. As a precaution, I now always carry a couple of salt sachets in my backpack. It's important to be mindful of electrolyte imbalances during exercise and strenuous activities, especially in warmer conditions.

'Mastering your migraine triggers will require perseverance and diligence, as you become more aware of how your body interacts with food, daily activities, and the environment.'

A major factor I have yet to mention is the food-related trigger. These triggers can be incredibly complex and challenging to identify due to the broad variety of potential trigger foods and the individualised nature of reactions. Several factors make pinpointing food triggers challenging. Firstly, they can vary significantly from person to person. Some individuals are highly sensitive to specific foods and may experience migraine attacks even with small amounts, while others are less sensitive and only develop symptoms when consuming larger quantities.

Another challenge with food triggers is the delayed onset of symptoms, which may not appear until the next day or later, making it difficult to connect them to specific foods consumed earlier.

Additionally, trigger foods, or more accurately, trigger compounds, often hide in packaged and pre-made foods under different names or as part of a complex ingredients list, making them even harder to identify.

2.5 The Snowball Effect: Understanding the Workings of Migraine Triggers

Migraine triggers often synergistically contribute to a cumulative response akin to a snowball rolling downhill. Each trigger adds to the build-up, resulting in a more intense reaction. This can occur when a single food contains multiple types of triggers, such as tyramine, histamine and glutamate, or when a meal combines different foods with different triggers, leading to an additive and increasingly intense migraine response.

However, this snowball effect extends beyond food-related triggers. All types of triggers, including environmental, hormonal and lifestyle factors, can contribute to this cumulative response. Among these, stress is often one of the most potent triggers. Stress can prime the body's internal systems, making it more susceptible to food-based triggers. When these factors combine, the snowball effect gains momentum, resulting in a heightened migraine response. Certain triggers may have little effect on their own with no adverse outcome. However, when combined with other triggers, their impact may intensify progressively, leading to a migraine.

To understand the origins of triggers and their physiological responses in the body, it is essential to acquaint oneself with two distinct trigger categories. Firstly, the 'external triggers', which originate from sources such as diet, mood and the environment. Secondly, the 'internal triggers', which originate from within the body itself. The internal triggers are the physiological responses generated by external triggers and are intricately linked to one's metabolic processes. These processes are highly individual, involving factors such as electrolyte dynamics, hormonal influences, neurological and immune activity, and genetic and nutrient influences. Fundamentally, all external triggers depend on the internal triggers. This means that the internal triggers are the primary drivers of a migraine, whereas external triggers act as catalysts to initiate the internal trigger process.

'Making the unpredictable predictable.'

The treatment strategies are uniquely different for external and internal triggers, and understanding the distinction between the two is crucial for the effective treatment and management of migraines. External triggers are managed through preventative treatment strategies to minimise exposure, and this may involve lifestyle and dietary changes and environmental modifications to minimise their impact. The internal triggers require a more nuanced approach that considers the individual's metabolic intricacies and involves strategies aimed at reducing the body's sensitivities and managing the physiological responses they elicit.

> *'The treatment strategies are uniquely different for
> external and internal triggers.
> Understanding the distinction between the two is crucial for the
> effective treatment and management of migraines.'*

Brain Bites and Guided Strategies

1. The trigger phase is the first stage in the migraine process, during which physiological changes are set in motion without the individual being aware. Migraine triggers are diverse. Identifying which of these affect you personally is key to managing migraines effectively. Becoming familiar with these triggers can empower you to take proactive measures and reduce the frequency and severity of your migraines. A helpful starting point is to carefully review the extensive list of external and internal triggers outlined in Section 5.2, and the 'Trigger Foods List' in Section 5.3 of the Therapy Kit.

2. Susceptibility and Sensitivity – susceptibility relates to the likelihood of experiencing migraines in response to the number of triggers, while sensitivity refers to the degree of response once a trigger is encountered. Understanding these factors is crucial for managing migraine frequency and severity.

3. Sensitivity to migraines can be influenced by a myriad of factors, including frequent and chronic stress, underlying metabolic conditions or diseases, and exposure to triggers. This increased sensitivity often manifests as a heightened inflammatory response, which can exacerbate migraine symptoms. For a comprehensive list of sensitivity factors that can lead to migraines, please refer to Chapter 4.

4. External vs Internal Triggers - external triggers originate from sources including diet, lifestyle and environmental factors, while internal triggers are physiological responses generated by external triggers.

5. It's time to kickstart your personal food and symptoms journal to identify potential triggers. Refer to The Therapy Kit, Section 5.4, 'Migraine Diary', for guidance on how to make the most of this diary. This tool can help you track your food intake, symptoms, and patterns to help identify what may be triggering your migraines.

2.6 The Premonition Phase

The premonition phase, medically described as the prodrome phase, is a part of the migraine stage marking the point at which triggers have set in motion an inflammatory event, progressively involving the trigeminovascular system.

This phase is also your final opportunity to halt the impending migraine attack or, at the very least, alleviate its intensity. Unfortunately, the use of complementary medicine is often ineffective at this stage, as the biological processes involved are already well underway. That said, our inner workings during this initial phase vary greatly, and there are no strict rules on how best to approach it. However, it is during this critical juncture that reliance on pharmaceutical medication comes to the fore, and that's okay because it is a part of this treatment journey, and the first priority will always be to prevent or abort the migraine attack.

The premonition phase exhibits inconsistent and subtle characteristics revealed through delicate and understated symptoms that can be easily overlooked amidst the hustle of daily life. This makes it challenging to pinpoint specific signs and symptoms. Acquiring the skill to capture the nuanced and transient nature of these symptoms requires practice and patient notation in your migraine diary.

The symptoms of the premonitory phase differ between individuals and can typically begin hours to days before the onset of the migraine headache. For some, this phase may manifest with bold and unmistakable symptoms, while others may believe there are no discernible signs as they tend to be subtle and vague. The following list represents the common symptoms that reveal themselves during the premonition phase:

- Mood changes – this may be irritability, short-temperedness, despondent, depressed, or anxious, outbursts of anger, or rage.

- Excessive yawning – Sometimes the jaw can hurt from excessive yawning.

- Visual disturbances - experiencing visual disturbances such as shimmering, sickle, zigzag lines, fireworks or blind spots.

- Food cravings – especially alcoholic beverages or simple carbohydrates and sweets.

- Crawling skin – individuals describe this as though they have small bugs under the skin, or the same sensation as when you get goose bumps when you are cold or you're experiencing strong emotions such as fear or euphoria.

- Poor sleep, frequent waking and not feeling settled.

- Vivid dreams and nightmares – These can occur a few days before a pending migraine

- Sensitivity to light or loud sounds – these sensitivities can make you irritable.

- Odours – quite often these sensitivities can make you slightly nauseas or irritable.

- Sensitivity to wind – this can make you grumpy or irritable.

- Fatigue or unusually tired, often occurring after midday.

- Neck pain – also stiffness or tension in the neck and shoulders.

- Jaw pain and molar pain.

You will find that with patience and growing awareness, these subtle symptoms will become increasingly obvious. By noting them in your migraine diary, you can trace back through your entries to identify the possible triggers that may have initiated these premonition symptoms.

The premonition symptoms that I used to experience were transient in nature, which is not unusual and makes identifying them a bit more challenging. My symptoms would interchange and vary in expression. One of these symptoms was extreme tiredness, which would always occur around 4-5 pm. Around that same time, I could also become grumpy and irritated about silly things, and be quite contrary.

During my experimental phase, I discovered that mindful breathing could prevent my migraines. This technique helped shift my nervous system back to parasympathetic activity and improved tissue oxygenation. I regularly use mindful breathing to prevent morning headaches, particularly after waking from vivid dreams, a common premonition symptom for me. My other premonition symptoms were lower jaw pain, often with referred pain to my molars, and occasionally excessive yawning until my jaw hurt.

The most intriguing of my premonition symptoms was not physical but rather a distinct feeling, an almost imperceptible awareness of impending change, a feeling that can easily be dismissed without conscious attention. For me, this feeling of imminent change triggered a faint undercurrent of anxiety, which I instinctively associated with the onset of a migraine. I later discovered that some of my patients experienced this sensation as well.

Brain Bites and Guided Strategies

- The premonition phase is the first stage of a migraine episode and involves the trigeminovascular system. Recognising this phase is vital as it provides the final opportunity to prevent or alleviate the impending migraine attack.

- The characteristics of premonition symptoms are delicate and understated, varying with each migraine. Due to the transient and nuanced nature of these symptoms, it is advisable to record them in a migraine trigger diary.

- Reliance on pharmaceuticals is emphasised during this phase as it is most likely the only treatment that can abort a migraine.

- To make progress in this phase, it's crucial to keep a migraine diary to monitor your patterns and symptoms. Refer to Chapter 5, Section 5.4, for guidance in how to use the migraine diary.

2.7 The Headache Phase

The headache phase is the most dreaded part of a migraine episode, due to the severe symptoms of a throbbing pain and, for some, accompanying nausea. Once the headache phase is reached, there is little we can do to alleviate the symptoms and we must simply endure the experience. However, there is a lot we can learn from the headache phase by understanding the underlying mechanisms. In this chapter, I will elaborate on the nature of the biochemical pathways and the chemical compounds involved in this process. From a naturopathic perspective, this understanding helps to address the process from a preventative approach with the aim to regulate the stress response, reduce the sensitivity of the neurological pathways, and allow the body to adapt to internal and external environmental and lifestyle factors.

The pathophysiology of a migraine headache involves a hierarchy of biochemical events. Once a trigger initiates a neurogenic response, the resulting noxious signal alters neurotransmitter activity. This in turn sets off a cascade of inflammatory molecules that act on blood vessels and pain receptors. The recruitment and release of these inflammatory molecules occur in a region called the trigeminovascular system, situated in the cervical spine region, covering the first three vertebral bodies in the neck region. It covers an extensive collection of nerve tissue, including the primary trigeminal nerve branching out to the ophthalmic, maxillary, and mandibular nerves, with pain signals expanding across the neck to the upper and lower jaw, eyes, temples, and skull. The occipital nerve activates pain signals at the base of the skull, the scalp, behind the ears, and typically behind the eyes. Both nerve pathways will also perpetuate the headache pain to intracranial and extracranial arteries.

From a physiological perspective, neurotransmitters function as the central command hub, directing the intricate regulation of the trigeminovascular system, much like a launch pad. Together, they play a vital role in maintaining optimal brain function and safeguarding neurological wellbeing. The intricate system orchestrates a myriad of functions, including regulation of cerebrovascular blood flow, blood pressure and brain tissue oxygenation to maintain homeostasis. For the migraineur, this region exhibits abnormally heightened sensitivity and tends to magnify signals within the brain's self-regulating mechanism, leading to an exaggerated response.

The trigeminovascular system plays a central role in initiating the headache phase, serving as a significant pathway for the release of inflammatory molecules and the transmission of pain signals. These signals extend to different regions of the head and cerebrovascular tissue.[24]

During this period, the trigeminal and occipital nerves in the neck region are indicative of potential premonition symptoms, which may be subtle and not immediately recognized. You may discern signs such as tenderness or tiredness in the shoulder area, accompanied by subconscious gestures like rubbing the neck or the base of the skull to alleviate tension or discomfort. Additionally, aching in the jaw and molars is a frequent premonition. For more information on premonition symptoms, refer to Section 2.6, 'The Premonition Phase' in this chapter.

The premonition symptoms are typically the beginnings of a trigeminal nerve 'sensitisation' and an indication that a migraine is looming. The incoming signals (noxious stimuli) from the trigger phase stimulate the release of several inflammatory mediators via the adenosine signalling pathway, including calcitonin gene related peptide (CGRP), substance P, glutamate, nitric oxide (NO), and mast cells, which release the additional inflammatory and vasodilatory mediators, histamine and prostaglandins.[25,26] These inflammatory molecules are discussed in the following section.

2.8 The Role of Neurotransmitters in Migraine Pain

Throughout this book, you'll frequently encounter discussions about the neurotransmitter, serotonin. That is because serotonin plays a central role in determining whether a migraine occurs or not. Serotonin is at the top of the hierarchy as a regulatory molecule, and optimal serotonin levels are crucial for regulating various inflammatory compounds associated with migraines, effectively keeping them in check. A drop in serotonin levels can lead to various physiological and psychological effects. In the nervous system, low serotonin levels are associated with mood disorders such as depression and anxiety. Serotonin is often referred to as the 'feel-good' neurotransmitter because it helps regulate mood, emotions and sleep-wake cycles. A decrease in serotonin can contribute to feelings of sadness, irritability and fatigue, as well as disruptions in sleep patterns. Monitoring these symptoms can serve as a gauge for serotonin levels, indicating a need for intervention. These symptoms can act as both triggers and premonition symptoms, and highlight the importance of early recognition and management.

In the immune system, serotonin plays a role in regulating inflammation. A drop in serotonin levels can lead to an increase in inflammatory responses, which will exacerbate conditions such as migraines. Serotonin also plays a role in regulating appetite and digestion. A decrease in serotonin levels may result in changes in appetite and gastrointestinal function, which are also common pre-migraine symptoms. Suboptimal serotonin levels can have widespread effects on both physical and mental health, as well as an increased susceptibility to migraines. For more information on serotonin, read Section 4.6, Chapter 4.

Let's take a closer look at the inflammatory compounds released when serotonin levels are suboptimal, and what leads to migraine pain. Serotonin plays a crucial role in how we perceive pain, with its levels fluctuating throughout the day. Generally, serotonin levels are higher during the day and lower at night. This daily variation can influence our sensitivity to pain. Lower nighttime serotonin contributes to an increased pain sensitivity. This could explain why pain often feels more intense in the evening and at night, affecting sleep quality. Additionally, the drop in serotonin at night may also be a factor in the onset of early morning migraines.

Now that we know the circadian rhythm affects serotonin levels, the question is: what other factors influence optimal brain serotonin? First, we need to consider nutrient deficiencies that impact the production of the serotonin pathway. The key amino acid precursor is tryptophan. However, there is competition between tissues for tryptophan, and if levels are insufficient, it is likely prioritised by the digestive system, leaving the brain wanting.

Other nutrients to consider are B6 and magnesium. A deficiency inhibits the function of the enzyme tryptophan hydroxylase in the conversion of tryptophan to 5-hydroxytryptophan (5-HTP) in the serotonin pathway. Tryptophan hydroxylase can also be inhibited by other factors such as inflammation, stress, insulin resistance (blood sugar dysregulation), and high doses of supplementary tryptophan.[27]

If serotonin production is inhibited due to the factors mentioned above tryptophan will be redirected through the kynurenine pathway to generate other important molecules. Consequently, this depletes tryptophan levels in brain tissue. Additionally, the increase in blood kynurenine inhibits tryptophan transport into the brain, further limiting its availability for 5-HTP and serotonin production.[27]

While serotonin is the primary neurotransmitter acting as a pain inhibitor, suboptimal levels of serotonin diminish the body's natural pain relief mechanisms, leading to the release of other pain-stimulating compounds. This process is activated through the trigeminovascular system, which involves specialised nerve endings called nociceptors that detect potential harm by stimulating pain.

The molecules that activate these nociceptors include well-known vasoactive substances such as CGRP, glutamate, substance P, histamine, and nitric oxide, which collectively enhance sensitivity and induce pain in cerebral blood vessels and cranial regions. The consequent constriction, dilation and stretching of blood vessels, typically observed during headache pathology, is a contributing factor to the sensation of pain.[28]

CGRP stands out as the most potent among vasodilators, and the most enduring in migraine pain. It is released from nerve fibres in the trigeminovascular system and nerve fibres covering the meningeal and cerebral blood vessels.

CGRPs' activity is also associated with other vasoactive compounds like nitric oxide and histamine. CGRP was discovered to be significantly elevated in both blood and saliva not only during an acute migraine attack, but also between migraine attacks with individuals suffering from chronic migraines.[25] Optimal serotonin levels inhibit CGRP activity; however, when physical or mental stressors present and serotonin levels drop, it leads to a rise in CGRP activity. In the 1990s, a migraine medication entered the market as a serotonin receptor agonist, collectively known as triptans, with the purpose of alleviating migraine headache pain. These drugs actively bind to serotonin receptors and have been shown to reduce serum levels of CGRP.[29] If you would like to know more about triptans and other pharmaceutical migraine medication, turn to Chapter 1 'What doctors don't tell you'.

Another compound involved in migraine pain is the neuropeptide substance P, which is the primary pain molecule that then acts on the Neurokinin-1 receptor (NK1 receptor). The substance P and NK1 receptor relationship plays an important role in neuroinflammation and the sensation of pain. Many of these receptors are present in the endothelium of cerebral blood vessels and their transmission works closely in conjunction with two other vasodilatory compounds, namely nitric oxide and CGRP.[30]

Substance P also contributes to the dilation of blood vessels and the recruitment of immune cells such as mediation of mast cells to release histamine, bradykinin and nitric oxide, which all contribute to the sensation of pain.[30]

Both substance P and glutamate, along with their receptors, prompted great interest among scientists for the development of a drug to halt the transmission of pain. However, this was not successful due to the complexity of the molecules and their diverse functions throughout the body, which resulted in undesirable side effects.

Several NK1 receptor antagonists were trialled for migraine treatment but proved unsuccessful.[31] However, the unexpected outcome led to the development of an antiemetic drug that prevents nausea and vomiting. This drug works by inhibiting substance P activity on the NK1 receptor in the brain, which controls the sensation of nausea and vomiting (emesis).

Another major player in the trigeminovascular pathway and its intricate network of molecular interactions, is adenosine, which plays a pivotal role in expressing CGRP through the adenosine receptors pathway. However, like most tissue receptors, there are many subtype receptors for various biological effects. The adenosine signalling pathway is no exception. Adenosine is involved in the regulation of the trigeminovascular system and is a key player in migraine pathophysiology. Adenosine levels witness a significant surge during stress responses, particularly during a migraine attack.[32] It is noteworthy to mention that elevated adenosine levels are directly involved in reducing serotonin levels through increased platelet uptake.[32] This leaves CGRP, glutamate, substance P, and other inflammatory compounds unopposed, leading to vascular dysregulation and consequently, a migraine headache. The surge in adenosine levels during stress reflects its role as a versatile molecule that participates in complex regulatory pathways to help the body adapt to challenging conditions. During a migraine episode, the exaggerated activity of this function contributes to the neurological and vascular changes associated with migraine symptoms.

Regulating the adenosine pathway is crucial in reducing the frequency and severity of migraines. Possible enzyme deficiency of adenosine deaminase allows raised tissue levels of adenosine and subsequent increased inflammation and sensitivity to migraines. The cofactor for adenosine deaminase production is zinc, an essential trace element, which has been shown to be deficient in migraine sufferers.[33,34] Zinc is also an important immune regulator, antioxidant and anti-inflammatory agent.[35] Another beneficial compound in regulating adenosine activity is the flavonoid, quercetin. This antioxidant compound plays a major role in immune regulation and has been shown to reduce high levels of adenosine.[36] Caffeine is also a notable inhibitor of adenosine activity and can alleviate migraine headache.

Brain Bites and Guided Strategies

- Serotonin plays a central role in migraine regulation, affecting mood, inflammation and pain perception. Low serotonin levels are associated with increased susceptibility to migraines.

- Symptoms such as mood changes, disrupted sleep and appetite alterations can indicate low serotonin levels.

- Inflammatory compounds like CGRP, substance P, glutamate, and histamine are released and contribute to migraine pain when serotonin levels are low.

The following strategies and treatments to reduce elevated adenosine levels and regulate the adenosine pathway can be found in Chapter 5, The Therapy Kit. Refer to the specified sections for the following:

- 'Stress Relief Strategies' – Go to Section 5.8. and following the subsections.

- Coffee, the potent adenosine receptor inhibitor – Go to Chapter 3, Section 3.12, 'A Delicious Dilemma'.

- Improving Zinc Status – Go to Subsection 5.7.3.

- Optimal dietary Quercetin and other antioxidants – You will find information on this in Subsection 5.8.3, 'Feed Your Stress'.

- Optimal 5-HTP and serotonin in brain tissue – Go to Subsection 5.7.1, '5-HTP', and Subsection 5.7.2, 'Magnesium'.

2.9 The Recovery Phase

The recovery phase is the final stage of a migraine episode, characterised by a range of symptoms and duration depending on the severity of the migraine attack and the type of medication taken. It is medically described as the postdrome phase, which basically means the set of symptoms after the migraine attack. For some, this phase is much like a hangover due to its association with feelings of fatigue and other lingering symptoms, similar to how one might feel after overindulgence in alcohol consumption.

While symptoms vary significantly among individuals, for me, it was the relief phase when the intense pain and torment had subsided, allowing me to finally fall into a restorative slumber. My primary symptom manifested as major fatigue, akin to having completed a marathon. I would have cravings for sour foods, salads, or soups, particularly vegetable soup. Additionally, I endured constipation and digestive issues in the subsequent days as a result of the diarrhoea and vomiting, and the occasional tachycardia due to a loss of body fluids and electrolytes.

Some of the more common symptoms during the recovery phase include fatigue, tiredness, mood swings, irritability, and feelings of depression. Some individuals may experience difficulty in concentration, or have generalised body aches, stiffness or muscle soreness. Digestive issues, such as constipation, bloating and digestive discomfort after eating, are typically a follow-up from vomiting and diarrhoea after a migraine episode. Hunger and cravings are also prevalent in this stage.

The recovery phase generally resolves within 24 hours, but for some individuals, particularly those who experienced vomiting and diarrhoea during the headache phase, may take longer to recover. Excessive vomiting can disrupt the delicate pH balance in the stomach, as it triggers the regurgitation of bile into both the stomach and the oesophagus through the vomiting reflex.

The discomfort may manifest as bloating, fullness, abdominal pain, or a general sense of unease in the digestive system. Restoring digestive balance is a gradual process that takes time.

Recovering from a migraine episode requires both time and patience as it's essential to listen to your body and respond to its needs. Rest and relaxation are key. Give yourself time to recover by getting adequate rest; sleep can be particularly beneficial during this phase. Hydration should be your next priority. Dehydration can trigger migraines, so make sure to drink plenty of water to rehydrate yourself. Once you're ready to get up, consider some gentle exercises. Engaging in light, gentle physical activities such as walking or stretching can help restore neurotransmitters. Depending on your appetite or if you are experiencing digestive symptoms, consider eating smaller, more frequent nutritious meals and opt for easily digestible foods, while practicing mindful eating habits. Importantly, manage your stress with stress-reducing techniques.

Addressing and managing stress may involve addressing any feelings of guilt that arise when you find yourself unwell at home. This is a common experience for individuals dealing with migraines. The inability to fulfill responsibilities and the need to rely on others. Friends, family, may trigger feelings of guilt as you are not able to fulfill social responsibilities and you feel that you are letting others down.

We can also feel guilty about missed opportunities and financial concerns. We all know that migraines can strike unexpectedly, causing you to miss out on planned events, social gatherings or important occasions. This can lead to a sense of guilt or stress for not being able to participate or cover your commitments.

We all have experienced that migraines can lead to missed workdays, potentially impacting one's income. The financial implications of frequent migraine attacks may contribute to guilt, especially if you feel responsible for the financial wellbeing of yourself and your family.

Migraines can be difficult for others to understand as the pain is invisible, and you may feel guilty when you struggle to effectively communicate the severity of your condition to those who may not fully grasp the impact it has on your daily life.

It is important for individuals with migraines to communicate openly with their support network, seek understanding from those around them, and work together to find ways to manage the condition effectively. Professional help, such as consulting with a healthcare provider or a mental health professional, can also be beneficial in addressing the emotional aspects of living with migraines.

Brain Bites and Guided Strategies

1. The recovery phase involves understanding symptoms, managing physical and emotional aspects, and prioritising self-care.

2. Recommendations for recovery include rest, adequate sleep, hydration, gentle exercises, and small, easily digestible, nutritious meals. Make sure you address electrolyte imbalance, dehydration and digestive capacity.

3. To manage your stress, refer to 'Stress Relief Strategies' Chapter 5, Section 5.8.

4. For emotional support, I encourage you to seek professional help through your health practitioner.

CHAPTER 3

The Origins of Migraine Triggers

3.1 Navigating the Realm of Foods and their Migraine Triggers

In this chapter, we will explore the presence and impact of three specific compounds that can lead to various food-related migraine triggers, specifically tyramine, histamine and glutamate. These compounds are commonly found in high-protein foods such as meats, seafood and dairy products, as well as in certain vegetables, nuts, seeds, and legumes. They are also naturally produced in the body for various biological functions. However, when their concentration exceeds the body's biological needs, these compounds can lead to adverse reactions such as headaches, rashes, nausea, and changes in blood pressure. While certain fresh produce like fruit and vegetables generally contain these compounds at low levels, factors such as food processing methods, cooking times, and storage conditions can significantly increase their concentrations.

Tyramine and histamine are formed through the breakdown (decarboxylation) of the amino acids tyrosine and histidine, respectively. Tyramine is a potent vasoconstrictor that can lead to symptoms of hypertension and headaches, while histamine acts as both a vasodilator and vasoconstrictor, depending on the type of receptor it activates.

Both tyramine and histamine, along with glutamate, can activate additional inflammatory and vasoactive compounds in the body, which can exacerbate the migraine process.

In the following sections of this chapter, I will reveal these three compounds in great depth, exploring both their sources and their impacts on health, as well as effective strategies for managing their intake.

3.2 Amines in foods: the hidden culprits

In foods, the amines histamine and tyramine are primarily produced as by-products of microbial activity, including that of lactic acid bacteria, which play a crucial role in the fermentation process.

These amines present in a variety of foods, especially high-protein foods like meats, seafood and dairy products, but also in certain vegetables, nuts and seeds and legumes.

It has long been established that high concentrations of food-based tyramine and histamine are toxic. As a result, the food industry adheres to strict guidelines during food processing, especially during fermentation of food products, to ensure safe levels of these amines. Yet, it is not uncommon for mild toxic levels of tyramine to be reached in fermented foods like cheeses and cured meats.[37]

For individuals sensitised to these compounds, even minor changes in amine concentrations can lead to adverse reactions. Common symptoms of high levels of tyramine include headache, rashes, tachycardia, nausea, and blood pressure variations due to the constriction or dilation of blood vessels.[38]

Tyramine and histamine are often present in the same foods, but there are exceptions. For example, tyramine is found in more foods compared to histamine, but generally at much lower concentrations. Avocado and plums are the only two fruits that contain tyramine.[39]

There is only a handful of fresh produce containing concerning levels of histamine and those include tomatoes, asparagus, spinach, aubergine, and avocado.

The concentration of amines can vary significantly, primarily depending on the freshness and storage duration of the products. Determining this in supermarket produce can be challenging, as many fruits and vegetables remain in controlled storage for weeks or even months before they end up in your shopping cart. In contrast to commercially processed foods, amine levels tend to be notably higher due to production methods and storage practices.

Amines are produced during various food processing methods, including heating during cooking and fermentation. Factors like moisture significantly influence amine levels in food. For example, fresh seafood, when grilled or fried, tends to have higher histamine concentrations compared to when it is raw or steamed.[40]

Among these processes, fermentation plays a key role in amine production, particularly in foods such as cheese, wine, cured meats, and the preparation of condiments such as fish sauce, soy sauce, and tomato sauce (ketchup). The fermentation process not only enhances the texture and flavour of these foods but also contributes to increased amine formation due to the denaturing of proteins.

Cheeses undergo a fermentation process in a controlled environment, referred to as aging or maturation. During this process, amines are naturally produced, with the amount of amine production dependent on both the cheese's protein content and the duration of the aging process.

Hard cheeses like cheddar, parmesan, and similar varieties contain high levels of protein, and therefore more amine production as the cheeses age. When selecting a hard cheese, it's advisable to choose a milder variety like cheddar that has been aged for 1-3 months or semi-matured for 3-6 months. It's best to avoid cheeses that have been aged for between 6 to 24 months. These are often referred to as 'tasty' or 'vintage' cheeses.

When it comes to international cheeses, with examples like the French Comte, the Swiss Emmental or Gruyere, or the Dutch Gouda cheese, the same principles apply. Different countries and regions can vary in their cheese aging processes. For example, aged Dutch or Swiss Emmental or Gruyere are typically high in protein and can have elevated amine levels. Italian Parmigiano-Reggiano and Spanish Manchego also follow this trend, with longer-aged varieties having higher amine content.

If you're concerned about amines but love cheese, it's a good idea to research specific international varieties to better understand their aging process and protein content. As a general rule, younger or less matured cheeses tend to have lower amine levels.

Soft cheeses such as Brie and Camembert contain lower protein levels and, consequently, lower concentrations of amines. However, their amine content can still vary depending on maturity, which is not always easy to determine from packaging alone. One useful indicator is the asking price. The longer a cheese is aged, the higher its cost. This principle also applies to cured meats such as prosciutto, ham, bacon, salami, and similar products.

Amines are present in non-fermented foods, including seafood, meats and various food preparation methods. These compounds will be formed during processes such as mincing, microwave cooking, boiling, and high-heat cooking. Be mindful when preparing foods like meat stews or bone broth, as amine levels increase with extended cooking times; the longer they cook, the higher the concentrations. Amine levels can also rise in leftover foods, so take care when storing home-cooked meals and takeout, as they will continue to increase as the food deteriorates. Additionally, packaged and canned foods, such as fish, legumes and dried meats, will also contain amines.

Initially, you will find it challenging to determine which amine or glutamate is responsible given that these foods typically contain a mix of these trigger compounds. Nevertheless, there are some food exceptions that will aid in pinpointing the various types involved.

As you make progress with your migraine diary, you will gradually develop the ability to identify your sensitivities to specific foods. This knowledge will empower you to select your meals with increased confidence.

Remember that these sensitivities can vary from person to person, which means you will have to do your own exploration to ascertain your reactions to various types and quantities of foods.

A detailed list of glutamate and amine-rich foods is available in 'The Therapy Kit', Chapter 5. Section 5.3, titled 'List of Top Foods that can Trigger Migraines'.

If you find that you have certain food sensitivities and you have begun to make discerning food choices, you will quickly see improvements in your migraine frequency.

But don't be deceived. Learning to understand the types of foods and quantity you can eat is a journey, and the best way to keep track of this is to start a migraine diary, which is covered in Section 5.4.

3.3 Amines and the Role of Gut Bacteria

While many are familiar with the presence of amines in foods, there's a general lack of awareness regarding the intricate regulation of these compounds within the gut and other parts of the body, including the brain. In the digestive system, the gut microbiome forms a vast community of bacteria crucial for optimal digestive function and numerous other essential effects throughout the body.

One significant role of the microbiome is the regulation of tyramine and histamine levels. Various bacterial strains are responsible for producing and degrading these amines.[41] Therefore, a healthy microbiome plays a crucial role in maintaining balanced levels of these compounds. However, changes in microbial composition, known as microbial dysbiosis, can disrupt this balance. This disruption can lead to increased concentrations of both tyramine and histamine in the body.

Microbial dysbiosis is a widespread gut disorder in modern society, often resulting in various digestive issues like reflux, food sensitivities, and intolerances. When chronic, it can contribute to the development of several diseases, including diabetes, obesity, cardiovascular disease, and allergies.[42]

In a healthy digestive system, the robust gut microbiome plays a crucial role in controlling the potential toxic effects of amines. This intricate regulation is facilitated by both the gut bacteria and specialised enzymes such as monoamine oxidase (MAO) and diamine oxidase (DAO). In the following sections, I will delve into more detailed information on how histamine and tyramine levels are regulated through these physiological processes.

3.4 The Histamine Trigger

Impaired histamine metabolism warrants careful consideration as a pivotal factor in the etiology of migraine pathology. The equilibrium between histamine production and degradation is delicate, and a disruption can lead to elevated histamine concentrations that can instigate a wide spectrum of pathological conditions that can affect multiple body systems.

It's widely understood that histamine can trigger allergy symptoms like hay fever. However, it's less known that this connection often arises from an imbalance in gut health. Equally, a dysregulation of histamine levels within the digestive system can result in typical gastrointestinal issues like cramping, bloating, constipation, and diarrhoea. Additionally, this imbalance can cause broader systemic symptoms like skin rashes, flushing, muscular pain, and fatigue. Despite these potential effects, mild disruptions in histamine levels within the digestive system may not always be immediately apparent.

Histamine is integral for digestive and immune function,[43] and its expression via many available mucosal mast cells is plentiful all along the digestive tract. Equally, there are many species of gut bacteria which produce and degrade histamine as an immune protective mechanism within the gut mucosa.[44,45]

A dysregulation of histamine can typically occur with digestive problems such as infections, inflammatory diseases, food allergies, and chronic food sensitivities. This pathological picture is mostly observed in a disparity between elevated histamine concentrations and a deficiency in histamine degrading enzymes, which can lead to histamine intolerance (histaminosis).

Individuals with histamine intolerance usually exhibit microbial dysbiosis, an imbalance in the community of gut bacteria and typically characterised by an abundance of histamine-secreting bacteria.[46] While it is commonly assumed that histamine intolerance is solely due to a deficiency in the diamine oxidase enzyme (DAO), this view oversimplifies the condition. There are cases of histamine intolerance where individuals have normal levels of DAO but exhibit marked gut dysbiosis and an abundance of histamine-secreting bacteria.[46]

Nevertheless, DAO is the principal histamine-degrading enzyme in the digestive system. It is an enzyme that is expressed in high concentrations in the upper intestinal enterocytes within the mucosal lining, where they are constantly released into the gut and bloodstream during digestion.[47] Impaired DAO activity will allow an increase in histamine absorption and consequently elevated blood histamine concentration. Maintaining histamine homeostasis relies on the delicate interplay between DAO enzyme activity and an optimal population of histamine-degrading bacteria.

Another key enzyme responsible for degrading and regulating histamine is Histamine N-methyltransferase (HNMT). Unlike DAO, which primarily functions in the gut, HNMT is more broadly expressed within cells and is particularly prominent in brain tissue. This localisation is not surprising, given that histamine receptors, which are crucial for neurological health, are widely distributed throughout cerebral tissue.

Polymorphic variations in the HNMT enzyme may influence the efficiency of histamine degradation in brain tissue.[48] The presence of polymorphic enzymes means that different individuals may have slightly different versions of the same enzyme, which can affect how they process histamine in the body.

Before we explore the dysregulation of histamine in cerebral tissue further, it's important to understand that dietary histamine cannot directly trigger a migraine because it cannot cross into brain tissue. The brain's biochemistry operates independently from the rest of the body and is highly selective about what substances it allows to enter through the semi-permeable membrane known as the blood-brain barrier. Histamine is one of the compounds that cannot pass through this barrier.

Although research shows that dietary histamine can impact migraines, the exact relationship is not fully understood. Studies have found that blood histamine levels rise during migraine episodes. Furthermore, research that involved the systemic administration of histamine consistently triggered and worsened headaches. These studies have also noted that people with migraines are more susceptible to histamine-induced headaches, which often developed into a full-blown migraine.[49,50,51]

The most likely scenario how dietary histamine induces a migraine is orchestrated through a neurological process facilitated by the trigeminovascular system, a regional connection point of sensory nerve cells, acting as the principal pathway for transmitting pain signals to the head and cerebral blood vessels. Subsequently, this inflammatory pathway can progress further by engaging histamine receptors within cerebral tissue, releasing additional inflammatory molecules that culminate in the onset of a migraine attack.

The role of histamine in body tissues becomes more complex due to the presence of multiple histamine receptors, of which four have been identified, all present in brain tissue. However, their intricate role in brain function and different patterns of interaction between histamine receptors and other neurotransmitters is highly complex and still largely unexplored.

All histamine receptors play a role in immune regulation including histamine 3 receptor (H3R), which stands out from the bunch as it is exclusive to brain tissue and the central nervous system with a high density in receptor numbers throughout the brain regions of the hippocampus, basal ganglia and cortex.

What is even more unique about this receptor is that unlike the other histamine receptors who are proactive in the inflammatory process, the H3 receptor has the ability to directly inhibit the release of histamine from neurons and mast cells in brain tissue.[51] This provides a regulatory mechanism to control histamine levels in the brain. Therefore, if the brain tightly regulates histamine levels via the H3 receptor, it is less susceptible to an inflammatory event. However, not everyone has optimal H3 receptor numbers and it is speculated that individuals with suboptimal numbers of the H3 receptor are more likely to suffer from headache and migraine pain.[51]

One of the reasons why some of us may have an inadequate number of these receptors is because certain polymorphic variants, such as A280V, in the H3 receptor gene can lead to reduced receptor expression of function in cerebral tissue.[52] This diminished activity allows histamine to rise and consequently increases susceptibility to migraine headaches.

From a therapeutic perspective, options for increasing the number of H3 receptors are limited. However, managing dietary histamine and digestive histamine production can help prevent H3 receptors from becoming overburdened, making it a recommended approach.

An increased concentration of histamine can also suggest an abnormally high mast cell expression. Histamine intolerance may well be the basis of abnormal mast cell expression and an escalated release of chemical mediators, which is a condition clinically referred to as mast cell activation syndrome (MCAS). Frequent or chronic digestive disturbances can upregulate mast cells and increase their sensitivity to any inflammatory response. This process is referred to as 'mast cell sensitisation'. When mast cells are exposed to certain triggers such as allergens or pathogens, they can undergo changes that make them more responsive to subsequent inflammatory signals. This heightened sensitivity can lead to an exaggerated release of inflammatory mediators like histamine, potentially worsening inflammatory conditions such as migraines.

The complexity of elevated histamine doesn't stop there; the activity of the principal histamine degrading enzyme DAO can be disrupted in more than one way. During inflammation, the mucosal enterocytes are prone to damage and directly affect the production of DAO.[39] Chronic digestive conditions like Irritable Bowel Disease[39] and celiac disease[53] are typical examples of mucosal damage. Inflammation of the digestive tract leads to more histamine production and inadequate DAO to regulate histamine levels.

Histamine also has competition with two other amines that rely on DAO for degradation, namely putrescine and spermidine. The presence of these dietary amines can potentially interfere with histamine levels. Small amounts of putrescine are found in most fruit and nuts with a high content in bananas, mushrooms, soybeans, passionfruit, pistachio, and citrus fruit. Extremely high levels of putrescine can be found in peas, corn and green peppers.

Keep in mind that amine levels can vary greatly in these foods and is dependent on their freshness, storage and processing. A good example is citrus fruit juices, which contain particularly high levels of putrescine, especially commercial orange, grapefruit and mandarin juices.[39] It is not unusual that high putrescine foods can mimic symptoms of histamine intolerance.

Several pharmaceutical drugs inhibit DAO activity. The antibiotic Clavulanic acid and antimalaria drug Chloroquine are potent inhibitors, reducing DAO activity by over 90%.[54] The high blood pressure medication Verapamil and Cimetidine for gastric acid reduction can inhibit DAO by 50%. Moderate inhibitors, reducing activity by just over 20%, include Metamizole for pain and fever, and the tricyclic antidepressant Amitriptyline. Less potent inhibitors, reducing activity by less than 20%, include Metoclopramide, a dopamine antagonist used for migraine and gastrointestinal issues, and Diclofenac, a non-steroidal anti-inflammatory drug.[54]

According to a couple of studies, thiamine (vitamin B1) has also been identified as an inhibitor of DAO,[47,54] but there is no explanation as to how the vitamin influences this inhibition. Nonetheless, this should be taken into consideration, particularly if you are using a multivitamin supplement. It's worth noting though, that the inhibitory capacity of thiamine is less than 20%.[54]

Brain Bites and Guided Strategies

- Impaired histamine metabolism is a result from factors such as gut dysbiosis, DAO deficiency, inflammation of the gut mucosa, competing amines including putrescine and spermidine, medication, genetic variants of the H3 receptor, and overactive mast cells.

- Vitamin B1 can inhibit DAO. Although the impact is relatively minor and may not significantly affect histamine metabolism, it is important to consider the cumulative effect of the different factors that reduce DAO activity.

Polymorphic variations in the HNMT enzyme may influence the efficiency of histamine degradation in brain tissue.

The following therapeutic interventions, available in The Therapy Kit in Chapter 5, contribute to the regulation of histamine levels.

1. To regulate dietary histamine, refer to the 'Amines and Glutamate protocol', Section 5.13.

2. To address dysbiosis, refer to 'Striving for Optimal Gut Health', Section 5.10.

3. To modulate mast cells activity, refer to 'Regulating Mast Cells', Chapter 5, Section 5.12.

4. Increasing the production of DAO activity, Chapter 5, Section 5.13, under subheading 'Enhancing Enzymes'.

5. Polymorphic variations in the HNMT enzyme and H3 receptor require an indirect therapeutic approach focused on supporting and optimizing the methylation pathway, as outlined in Chapter 5, Section 5.11.

3.5 The Tyramine Trigger

Dietary tyramine is rapidly absorbed from the gut and degraded by the enzyme monoamine oxidase (MAO), which is the primary enzyme that helps to degrade several amines, including dopamine, serotonin, and norepinephrine.

Tyramine's physiological role in the body is still not clear, but we know that tyramine works on specific trace amine-associated receptors (TAAR), which are predominantly found in the central nervous system and brain. However, what is interesting is that the stomach and small intestine have a particularly large amount of TAAR receptors, which are suggested to play a role in the gut brain axis,[55] and which I speculate may have a relationship with cerebral vasoconstriction and the pathogenesis to headaches and migraine.

Both dietary and endogenous tyramine are regulated by the MAO enzyme system and an insufficient activity of MAO will lead to an increased exposure of tyramine.

Excess tyramine is further metabolised into octopamine, which also acts on TAAR receptors, causing vasoconstriction.[56] The body's response to high levels of tyramine will also activate the stress hormone norepinephrine which will further exacerbate vasoconstriction. This leads to common symptoms for susceptible individuals, including high blood pressure, nausea, headaches, and migraines.

Interestingly, studies have demonstrated that the plasma levels of tyramine, octopamine, noradrenaline, and dopamine are several times greater in chronic migraine sufferers when compared to healthy subjects with no headaches or migraines.[57]

There are several factors that influence MAO activity and tyramine degradation. Firstly, it is important to consider the impact of pharmaceutical drugs known as monoamine oxidase inhibitors (MAOIs), which are used for depression. Ideally, when prescribing MAOIs, practitioners should advise patients to avoid consuming high-tyramine foods to prevent adverse side effects on blood pressure. Similarly, individuals sensitive to tyramine are more likely to experience headaches and migraines.

Common brands of MAOIs include Nardil (phenelzine), Parnate tranylcypromine), Marplan (isocarboxazid) and Emsam (selegiline).

Another substance that functions as a MAO inhibitor is tobacco. Studies using brain imaging have shown that chronic smoking can lead to a notable reduction of MAO activity by 30-40%.[58] This should not only be considered by smokers but also by individuals who work or live in smoking environments.

An interesting aspect of tyramine is its pharmacokinetics, which is the movement and elimination of the amine within the body. Generally, dietary tyramine is readily absorbed and can be present in circulation within ten minutes of ingestion.[59] However, it's worthy to note that the authors mention significant variations in how dietary tyramine is metabolised across individuals, with some processing it more efficiently than others. Consequently, the key question revolves around understanding what might be causing the delay in tyramine degradation within the body, and I would speculate that some migraineurs metabolise tyramine less efficiently.

Previous studies have suggested that the disparity in the clearance rate of this amine may be attributed to genetic variants of both MAO and the organic cation transporter (OCT1), which play crucial roles in hepatic tissue by aiding in the elimination of tyramine. Despite these propositions, this hypothesis has not yet come to light.[59]

The epigenetics of an individual can directly influence enzyme production through DNA methylation and gene expression. Epigenetics encompasses various aspects of an individual's life, including stressors, lifestyle factors like nutrition and physical activity, and any underlying health conditions. Put simply, epigenetics can impact gene function by either switching them on or off.

According to a study, MAO activity varies widely within the population, suggesting a substantial influence of environmental and dietary factors on gene expression.[60] Addressing these epigenetic factors through nutrient assessment can improve DNA methylation and subsequently MAO activity.

Brain Bites and Guided Strategies

- Tyramine is rapidly absorbed from the gut and degraded by the enzyme monoamine oxidase (MAO), which also degrades dopamine, serotonin and norepinephrine. The enzyme can vary in metabolism efficiency among individuals, possibly contributing to migraine susceptibility.

- Tyramine acts on trace amine-associated receptors (TAAR) in the central nervous system and gut, potentially influencing the gut-brain axis and vasoconstriction related to headaches and consequential rebound migraine.

- Insufficient MAO and organic cation transporter (OCT1) activity can lead to increased tyramine exposure, which may contribute to symptoms like high blood pressure, nausea, headaches, and migraines.

- MAO inhibitors (MAOIs) used for depression can increase sensitivity to tyramine, leading to potential adverse effects on blood pressure. Tobacco can also reduce MAO activity, potentially affecting tyramine metabolism.

- Epigenetic factors, including stress, nutrition, physical activity, and health conditions, can impact MAO enzyme activity.

To address epigenetic factors, nutrient deficiencies and tyramine absorption and metabolism, refer to the following strategies in The Therapy Kit.

1. 'Effective Treatment Strategies for Amines and Glutamate' – Chapter 5, Section 5.13

2. 'Striving for Optimal Gut Health' – Chapter 5, Section 5.10

3.6 The Pleiotropic Nature of Glutamate: The Master Neurotransmitter

The amino acid glutamate is primarily recognised as an excitatory neurotransmitter with various roles in the central nervous system, including crucial functions in brain development, learning and memory. Its involvement in migraines stems from its ability to regulate neurotransmitters like dopamine, serotonin and noradrenaline, as well as its role in releasing inflammatory compounds and transmitting pain signals in the brain. In essence, glutamate is the master neurotransmitter.

Despite its known role for migraine pathology in the brain, dietary glutamate is often overlooked as a trigger for migraine. There are three good reasons for this. Firstly, dietary glutamate cannot cross the blood brain barrier and therefore cannot directly affect brain glutamate levels.[61]

Secondly, current research is inconclusive and limited, with inadequate evidence to draw from, and current available evidence is insufficient due to limited samples in research participants. Lastly, human clinical trials will always have their limitations in establishing the cause of disease due to individual variability and the influence of their environment. The complex and multivariate nature of migraine exemplifies the challenges in understanding the causative factors of this disorder.

Nevertheless, the collection of clinical evidence suggests that dietary glutamate or abnormalities in glutamate signalling, including excessive release or impaired clearance of glutamate, may lead to increased neuronal excitability and contribute to the development of migraine attacks.

It has also been demonstrated that there are elevated glutamate levels in the brains of migraine sufferers, particularly during migraine attacks.[62]

Additionally, studies in rats have shown that increased levels of peripheral glutamate can lower the threshold for trigeminovascular neuron excitation and increase blood flow in the dura mater. This finding suggests that the dysregulation of the peripheral glutamatergic system may contribute to migraine pathogenesis,[63] potentially involving dietary sources of glutamate.

In the brain, migraine pain transmission occurs through the action of glutamate on the N-methyl-D-aspartate (NMDA) receptors, which are located peripherally around the trigeminovascular system. When these receptors are activated, inflammation and pain are triggered through the release of substance P and calcitonin gene-related peptide (CGRP).[64] Prolonged or frequent activation of these NMDA receptors can enhance the nervous system's sensitivity, leading to changes in synaptic plasticity. This refers to the ability of synapses to strengthen or weaken over time in response to activity. For a deeper understanding of brain plasticity, refer to Chapter 4, Section 4.4, 'A Matter of Brain Plasticity'.

3.7 Glutamate in Food - Umami

Glutamate levels vary significantly among different foods. While some plant-based foods naturally contain high amounts of glutamate, protein-based foods like meats, seafood and dairy products can have even higher levels. This is because glutamate is an amino acid, and amino acids are components of protein. Glutamate is particularly noteworthy among amino acids, with approximately 5-12 grams of glutamate per 100 grams of protein.[65]

Then there are the many processed foods which have additional glutamate additives in the form of monosodium glutamate (MSG), caseinate, gelatine, and other hidden forms of glutamate, which I will discuss in more detail a bit later in this chapter.

Additionally, much of the glutamate in foods is bound to protein with varying amounts as free glutamate. This discussion will primarily focus on the role of 'free glutamate' as a trigger for stimulating the neurological pathway in some migraine susceptible individuals. 'Glutamate' will be used as a reference term throughout this discussion.

The natural flavours of foods are significantly influenced by amino acids and although glutamate is no exception, it is one of the more unique amino acids that influences 'umami', regarded as the fifth primary taste in addition to salty, sweet, sour, and bitter.

Umami can be interpreted as 'tastiness' or 'deliciousness' and adds an extra dimension to the flavour of certain foods.[66] For centuries, foods like fermented condiments such as soy sauce and fish sauce have been used as primary flavouring agents. The unique flavour of umami also enhances foods like charcuterie, deli meats and cheeses through their fermentation and ageing processes.

You may recall the previous discussion on the fermentation and ageing process under the heading of 'Amines in Foods'. It is the same food preparation methods that will liberate glutamate. The fermentation and ageing of these foods encourage protein breakdown, resulting in the accumulation of free glutamate, which subsequently imparts the delightful umami taste.

Pork contains high levels of glutamate and histamine among animal proteins. This is due to the naturally high levels of histidine and glutamic acid in both the meat and fat of pork, which, during the preparation process, can lead to the production of glutamate and histamine.

I should also mention that beef contains a relatively high amount of glutamate, which is released during cooking—especially when minced or stewed. The increased levels of free glutamate, which range from approximately 10 to 20 mg per 100 grams of beef, can trigger migraines in some individuals. In contrast, lamb contains lower levels of free glutamate, around 5 to 10 mg per 100 grams. Several patients in my clinic regularly experienced migraines after consuming beef, but after switching to lamb, they reported a significant reduction in their symptoms. The exact glutamate content varies depending on factors such as the specific cut, preparation method, and cooking process. Since free glutamate is more likely to be released through mincing and stewing, beef tends to contribute more to dietary glutamate exposure than lamb.

Glutamate also occurs naturally in various fresh foods. Algae, tomatoes, mushrooms, hemp, and walnuts, for example, contain significant amounts of glutamate. The humble yet exceptionally versatile tomato, renowned for its rich umami flavour, owes its unique taste to its high glutamate content, particularly concentrated within the pulp of the fruit. This natural savouriness has made it a staple in tomato sauce-based dishes, as well as the popular condiment, ketchup.

Another common source of glutamate is monosodium glutamate (MSG), often listed as E621 on ingredient labels. Despite some controversy, MSG is widely used as a flavour enhancer in various cuisines, including Asian cooking, and is found in numerous processed and cooked foods. These include instant meals, frozen dishes, canned soups, sauces, snack foods, desserts, and even chocolates.

The Food Standards Australia New Zealand (FSANZ) and The US Food and Drug Administration (FDA) require that foods containing added MSG must list the ingredient for consumers to make informed choices. But MSG is often considered a controversial ingredient, and many people avoid it due to concerns about its potential health effects, which can be experienced with symptoms of headache, flushing, sweating, nausea, and tingling.

Needless to say, food manufacturers are well aware of this and have strategically changed the wording of MSG to obscure their use of glutamate from the public.

Finding a food label that explicitly lists 'monosodium glutamate' is a rare nowadays. Instead, you need to carefully scrutinise food labels for the terms 'flavouring', 'food additive 621' or 'flavour enhancer 621'.

MSG also comes in the form of Monopotassium Glutamate (E 622), Calcium Glutamate (E623) and Monoammonium Glutamate (E624). These are found in a range of processed foods, including chips, snacks, pizzas, ready cooked foods, olives, meat products, instant soups in sachets, and charcuterie meats.

You will also need to check food labels for other additives containing glutamate, such as gelatin, yeast extract, hydrolysed yeast, soy extract, hydrolysed milk, hydrolysed vegetable proteins, and protein isolate, which can contain up to 20% glutamate.

Lastly, calcium caseinate and sodium caseinate, which are highly processed milk proteins, contain a considerable amount of glutamate. These are often used in processed foods for their stabilising, emulsifying, and protein enhancing properties, in products such as processed cheese, protein shakes and bars, and baked goods such as cakes, cookies, and snack bars.

The extensive use of these additives highlights the importance of glutamate's ability to enhance the savory, umami taste in foods, making it a popular choice in many culinary applications.

Brain Bites and Guided Strategies

1. Glutamate is implicated in migraines due to its role in regulating neurotransmitters like dopamine, serotonin and noradrenaline, as well as its involvement in releasing inflammatory compounds and transmitting pain signals in the brain.

2. Glutamate acts on N-methyl-D-aspartate (NMDA) receptors in the brain, triggering inflammation and pain through the release of substance P and calcitonin gene-related peptide (CGRP).

3. Prolonged or frequent activation of NMDA receptors can enhance nervous system sensitivity, leading to changes in synaptic plasticity with more frequent and severe migraines.

4. Dietary glutamate is often overlooked as a trigger for migraines because it cannot cross the blood-brain barrier to directly affect brain glutamate levels. However, clinical evidence suggests that abnormalities in peripheral glutamate levels, potentially dietary glutamate, can contribute to increased neuronal excitability and the development of migraine attacks.

For glutamate sensitivity consider the following strategies:

1. **Dietary changes:** Free glutamate occurs naturally in many foods and is particularly high in fermented and processed foods. To become more acquainted with these foods, consult the 'List of Top Foods that can Trigger Migraines' in Chapter 5, Section 5.3.

2. **Food labels:** Since glutamate additives can appear under various names in processed foods, it is important to carefully check nutrition labels to spot any form of these additives. You will also find these listed in the 'List of Top Foods that can Trigger Migraines'.

3. **Stress management:** Stress has been shown to adversely affect the levels of tissue glutamate. For strategies to manage stress effectively, refer to the 'Stress Relief Strategies' in Chapter 5, Section 5.8.

4. **Nutritional support:** Magnesium can regulate glutamate activity. Refer to 'Magnesium' in Chapter 5, Subsection 5.7.2. Including under 'Effective Treatment Strategies for Amines and Glutamate' in Chapter 5, Section 5.13.

3.8 The Estrogen Connection: That Time of the Month Again

Following stress, hormone cyclic changes in women represent the second most frequent migraine trigger. These changes typically occur in the second half of the menstrual cycle, prior to menstruation. From a therapeutic perspective, and unlike any other triggers, managing hormonal triggers presents a significant challenge in migraine treatment, due to their inherent connection to the body's natural metabolic cycles. The cyclical effects of the hormones estrogen and progesterone can both trigger migraines and, conversely, contribute to their prevention.

The complexity of estrogen's influence on the body extends well beyond reproductive function, but the area that I found of particular interest is estrogen's profound relationship with serotonin and its influence on mood and immune regulation. Serotonin is a neurotransmitter involved in regulating mood, sleep and appetite, among other functions. As we now know, during a stressful event, serotonin levels can decline, potentially triggering a migraine. Similarly, during the luteal phase of the menstrual cycle, estrogen levels drop, leading to a decrease in serotonin levels, which can in turn trigger migraines in susceptible individuals.

Estrogen brings out the best in serotonin, promoting optimal serotonin synthesis and receptor function in brain tissue[67] The way estrogen does this is by reducing the activity of the monoamine oxidase enzyme, which plays a role in serotonin clearance.[68] Additionally, estrogen downregulates pain and inflammation via the reduction of glutamate activity, and downregulating the expression of the NMDA glutamate receptors.[69]

However, a decline in estrogen levels also promotes a decline in serotonin and leaves glutamate and other proinflammatory compounds unopposed. Estrogen's decline begins during the luteal phase, the second half of the menstrual cycle, before the start of menstruation. During this time the body is at its most vulnerable, and the drop in serotonin and dopamine triggers a subsequent increase in norepinephrine and other pro-inflammatory effects.[70]

The pro-inflammatory effects commonly observed in the symptoms of premenstrual tension (PMS), are characterised by heightened pain perception, which contributes to symptoms such as menstrual cramps and breast tenderness.

Additionally, the decrease in serotonin levels is associated with PMS symptoms such as mood swings, depression, fatigue, and insomnia. For some, the temporary hormone fluctuation, drop in serotonin, and increase in norepinephrine, leaves nitric oxide and CGRP unopposed. This leads to the activation of trigeminal nerve fibres, potentially making women more susceptible to migraine symptoms.[71]

During the luteal phase, progesterone levels rise to prepare the uterus for a potential pregnancy. In addition to this primary role, progesterone has a crucial function in dampening the immune response. This response is a critical mechanism designed to prevent an immune reaction towards sperm and a potential embryo, thereby facilitating the delicate balance required for reproductive processes.

It is this dampened immunity that potentially makes the body more susceptible to infections, some of which are more commonly seen during this part of the menstrual cycle, with herpes virus outbreaks and urinary infections among the most frequent.

The likelihood for women experiencing a migraine during this period is heightened as the body is at its most vulnerable. While it is essential to respect the natural hormonal cycle, there are specific areas that can be strategically addressed to enhance overall wellbeing.

A full dietary analysis will also help identify and correct any nutrient deficiencies.

This analysis can be expanded to assess the dietary intake of phytoestrogen rich foods and develop personalised dietary strategies to enhance their consumption and support hormonal balance. The naturally occurring plant compounds such as the isoflavones daidzein and genistein can bind to estrogen receptors and provide a mild estrogenic effect, potentially alleviating migraines. The best sources of these compounds are soybeans and soy-based products including tofu, soy milk, tempeh, and miso. On my website you will find more helpful information on natural phytoestrogen products and recipes.

Brain Bites and Guided Strategies

- Hormonal cyclic changes, especially in the latter half of the menstrual cycle, significantly trigger migraines in women. This is characterised by a decline in estrogen before menstruation, which is accompanied by a drop in serotonin levels, leading to increased susceptibility to migraines.

There are several strategies you can consider to reduce the susceptibility to migraines during this part of the menstrual cycle.

1. Reducing stress can improve hormone production, regulate the menstrual cycle and improve serotonin levels. Stress-reducing techniques can help mitigate this effect. Refer to 'Stress Relief Strategies', Chapter 5, Section 5.8.

2. To resolve any digestive issues and improve the gut bacteria, refer to 'Striving for Optimal Gut Function' in Chapter 5, Section 5.10.

3. To improve immunity and managing inflammatory conditions, refer to 'Regulating Mast Cells and Inflammation' in Chapter 5, Section 5.12.

4. Work with your practitioner to undertake a thorough dietary analysis to address any nutrient deficiencies. This process will help identify specific areas where your diet may be lacking, allowing you to make targeted changes to enhance your overall wellbeing.

3.9 Hypoglycemia

An abnormal drop in blood sugar (hypoglycemia) can be a potent migraine trigger, and there are numerous conditions and medications that can lead to this condition.

Typical symptoms of hypoglycemia can include hunger pains, unusual sweating, shakiness (typically in the hands and fingers), weakness with fatigue, irritability, anxiety, a rapid heartbeat, or headaches (which can lead to migraines in susceptible people). If any of these symptoms are a regular occurrence it is important to consult your healthcare practitioner to determine the cause of your hypoglycemia.

In this discussion, we will focus on non-diabetic hypoglycemia, which is characterised by an acute drop in blood sugar as the body is not efficiently producing glucose from other sources such as body fat or protein.

There are two common types of hypoglycemic events: reactive hypoglycemia and fasting hypoglycemia. Reactive hypoglycemia occurs when you don't eat in a timely manner, typically two to four hours after a meal. Whereas fasting hypoglycemia (deliberate fasting) occurs after approximately five to eight hours without food.

Regular production of glucose is crucial, especially when dietary and stored glucose is depleted. The brain, in particular, has a considerable energy requirement, with 25% of the body's glucose demand dedicated to fuelling its functions.[72] However, frequent consumption of simple carbohydrates in the diet can often lead to hypoglycemic events. During these events, the body craves instant sugars, which can be satisfied by consuming more simple carbohydrates. This instant gratification overrides the body's gluconeogenesis pathway, which is responsible for producing glucose from fats and proteins when needed. While this pathway requires more effort and energy, the body instinctively favours the easier option of consuming readily available sugars. Sugar cravings serve as a signal that the body is seeking an immediate energy source rather than engaging in the more complex process of glucose production.

Hypoglycemic episodes activate the body's sensitised stress response, leading to the release of inflammatory molecules as it strives to restore balance. This response induces an excitotoxic state in brain tissue, characterised by the release of glutamate. This sets off a cascade of other inflammatory mediators, with a vasoconstrictive induced headache and ultimately a rebound migraine.[73]

Brain Bites and Guided Strategies

- Hypoglycemia can be a potent trigger for migraines and commonly occurs with triggers such as deliberate fasting or skipping meals.

- Frequent consumption of simple carbohydrates can often result in recurring hypoglycemic episodes. To mitigate these events, it is essential to regulate blood sugar levels through dietary modifications and enhancing digestive function.

In The Therapy Kit, you will find the following strategies to helps restore blood sugar levels.

- 'Essential Tips for Maintaining Stable Blood Sugar Levels' – Chapter 5, Section 5.14.

- To enhance digestive function, refer to 'Striving for Optimal Gut Function' – Chapter 5, Section 5.10.

3.10 The Nitrate Connection

Nitrates are a relatively overlooked topic in migraine literature, but I firmly believe that nitrates derived from foods can be a potential migraine trigger through the production of nitric oxide, a compound which plays a significant role in the pathogenesis of migraines.

Nitric oxide and glutamate work closely together by activating pain receptors (nociceptors) and a follow up release of glutamate, substance P and calcitonin gene-related peptide (CGRP) through the trigeminovascular system.[74]

Nitrate and nitrites are naturally occurring compounds in many foods. However, in processed foods, especially cured meats like ham, bacon, luncheon meats, and sausages, nitrates are primarily used as additives, especially to enhance colour, but also for flavour and as an antimicrobial agent.

A couple of early studies from the 1970s focused on nitrates in processed meats and the cause of nitrate-sensitive headaches, which became the term 'the hot-dog headache'[75].

For some reason, these studies fell by the wayside, possibly due to better regulation of nitrates in these processed foods. Yet, nitrates in plant-based foods were never addressed, which is odd considering that approximately 80% of dietary nitrates are derived from vegetables.[76]

Plant-based foods, notably leafy greens like spinach, kale, lettuce, arugula, celery, and Chinese cabbage, are exceptionally rich in nitrates. Additionally, beetroot, watermelon and radish also have a significant nitrate content.[76] Watermelon appears to be a particularly common trigger, potentially due to higher levels of consumption of this fruit.[77,78]

Dietary nitrates are easily absorbed via salivary glands in the mouth and digestive system. Much of the nitrate (NO_3) is converted to nitrites (NO_2) by nitrate reducing bacteria both in the mouth and digestive system, with blood nitrite levels peaking in approximately three hours post ingestion. Once absorbed into the blood and in circulation, nitrites are converted into nitric oxide (NO). Dietary nitrates are stored in many types of tissue, including haemoglobin, and are a substantial contribution to the bioavailable pool for nitric oxide.[79]

The conversion of nitrites to nitric oxide within the body play subsequent diverse physiological functions, most notably as a vasodilator for blood pressure homeostasis.[76] However, the question arises of the potential impact of dietary nitrates in the migraine process. It is plausible that certain individuals afflicted with migraine exhibit a heightened susceptibility to dietary nitrates, which could potentially act as a catalyst in a snowball effect with other triggers.

It has been established that an excess of nitric oxide and its associated vasodilatory effects can trigger migraine-like headaches, which is a common side effect experienced by angina patients taking nitroglycerin. Research studies have consistently demonstrated that the administration of nitroglycerine in healthy subjects, resulted in the onset of throbbing headaches within a short duration.[80,81]

What is notable is that a double-blind study employing the same intravenous nitroglycerin method on migraine patients, revealed a significantly heightened sensitivity, resulting in a more intense and prolonged throbbing headache compared to individuals without migraine.[82] Furthermore, circulating nitrates have shown to be significantly higher during a migraine attack and drop back to normal levels during migraine free periods.[83]

There is strong evidence supporting the potential vasodilatory effects of dietary nitrates. Several studies have concluded that a diet rich in plant foods can increase blood nitric oxide (NO) levels and reduce blood pressure.[84-86] There is also potential relationship between the amount of vegetables people consume and its effect on the population of bacteria that reduce nitrates. This can lead to higher levels of dietary nitrites, which can then increase nitric oxide production. Interestingly, a separate study discovered that migraine patients tend to harbor a higher concentration of nitrate-reducing bacteria in their oral cavity compared to individuals who do not experience migraines.[87]

Streptococcus and *Pseudomonas* nitrate-reducing bacterial are the more dominant species in the oral cavity.[87] However, other nitrate-reducing bacteria are also present and include *Neisseria, Staphylococcus, Rothia, Haemophilus, Prevotella, Veillonella, and the Pasteurella* species.[88] Interestingly, the use of antibacterial mouthwash can substantially reduce blood nitrite levels. In other words, the elimination of nitrite producing bacteria appears to exert a direct influence on the nitric oxide pathway responsible for vasodilation.[89] Remarkably, the same intervention observed an increase in blood pressure in a group of hypertensive individuals using antibacterial mouthwash.[86]

Brain Bites and Guided Strategies

- Nitrates, found in both processed and natural foods, can potentially trigger migraines by producing nitric oxide. There is a potential link between dietary nitrates, nitric oxide production and migraine susceptibility,

- Certain individuals may be more sensitive to dietary nitrates, which could exacerbate migraine attacks, possibly acting as a catalyst in conjunction with other triggers.

- The population of bacteria in the oral cavity that reduces nitrates may impact nitric oxide production. Migraine patients tend to have higher concentrations of nitrate-reducing bacteria, which can be reduced by antibacterial mouthwash.

- To address nitrates, go to The Therapy Kit, under the heading 'Nitrates Strategies' in Chapter 5, Section 5.9.

3.11 Alcoholic Beverages: I'll Have a Mocktail Please!

Alcohol consumption is widely recognised for its propensity to induce tension headaches and the classic hangover. Large-scale, population based studies and clinical population studies have consistently demonstrated alcoholic beverages as a headache trigger in both migraine and non-migraine subjects.[95–97]

Alcoholic beverages are practically a cocktail of vasoactive molecules and should be enjoyed with great caution. Here is why. In the context of the nitrate and nitric oxide pathway we just explored, ethanol plays a significant role in the generation of nitric oxide. Most alcoholic beverages contain small amounts of nitrates and nitrites with the notable exception of beer. However, the connection between ethanol and nitric oxide lies not in the nitrate content but in the nitric oxide produced within the body during the metabolism of ethanol.

This process involves two significant metabolic steps associated with a vasodilatory effect. The first step occurs as ethanol reaches the blood stream and begins to affect the brain within minutes of initial alcoholic beverage consumption. Ethanol exerts a direct influence on the vascular walls to activate nitric oxide and consequential vasodilation.[90]

The vasodilatory effect is initiated through the Transient Receptor Potential Vanilloid 1 receptor (TRPV1). This receptor functions as a sensory monitor in the epithelial walls and reacts to any anomalies in the blood that it deems as noxious. The noxious stimuli triggers vasodilation, inflammation and pain through the release of inflammatory mediators such as nitric oxide and CGRP, which is the most potent vasodilator of all molecules.[91]

The second step of ethanol's metabolic fate is the production of acetaldehyde, a cytotoxic substance that also possesses potent vasodilatory properties. Acetaldehyde further triggers the synthesis of prostaglandin I2 (PGI2), a well-known inflammatory and vasodilatory mediator.[92]

Acetaldehyde is a normal metabolic product formed by the oxidation (breakdown) of ethanol, a process that also occurs in alcoholic beverages, with concentrations ranging from 50-100 mg/L. Sherry is known for the highest concentration of acetaldehyde, which contribute to its characteristic 'aldehydic' aromas.

The potent vasodilatory effect from ethanol and acetaldehyde is met with a surge of serotonin, which serves as a compensatory response to counteract the inordinate vasodilation.[93] The initial surge in serotonin levels is responsible for the feelings of euphoria and a sense of wellbeing induced by initial alcohol consumption. However, the benefit of increased serotonin is not to make the drinker feel good, rather, it serves as a vital homeostatic mechanism in promoting a vasoconstrictive effect.

Many alcoholic beverages also contain the vasoactive amines histamine and tyramine, as well as the amino acid glutamate, which collectively exert a significant influence on individuals who are susceptible to migraines.

Much like food processing, the ageing or fortifying of alcoholic beverages will increase the presence of these influential constituents. Red wines, for example, have more histamine and tyramine compared to white wine. Red wines also contain tannins, which are present as polyphenols in the skin and seeds of dark grapes. Tannins are described as dry, astringent and slightly bitter to the taste, contributing to the characteristic flavour of red wines. Generally, darker wines contain higher levels of tannins. Higher tannin content also suggests that the wine has aged longer, allowing more compounds to be extracted from the grape skins. This, in turn, leads to greater production of histamine and tyramine. Once a bottle is opened, the oxidation process continues, causing histamine and tyramine levels to steadily rise, and likewise, the risk of migraine.

The primary tannins which give red wine the distinctive astringency and bitterness are polyphenols called proanthocyanidins, well known for their antioxidant activity, but less known for their serotonin boosting activity. These polyphenolic compounds have the ability to increase serotonin levels by inhibiting the enzyme monoamine oxidase, which degrades serotonin.[94]

These three mechanisms collectively result in elevated serotonin levels, which may cause excessive vasoconstriction in cerebral tissue and trigger a tension-type headache. This vasoconstriction can set off a cascade effect, leading to an overactive rebound vasodilation as the body's homeostatic systems attempt to restore normal vascular function. This process can ultimately lead to a migraine.

It is likely that red wine's higher susceptibility to triggering migraines can be attributed to the three converging mechanisms: ethanol acting through the vanilloid 1 receptor; the generation of acetaldehyde; and the suppression of monoamine oxidase activity by the polyphenolic compounds, especially in red wines.

If you're a red wine lover looking to explore how much wine you can enjoy without triggering a migraine, paying attention to tannin levels can be a helpful guide in choosing wines. Lower-tannin wines may be less likely to provoke migraines, so experimenting with these could help you find options that suit you best. But keep in mind that ethanol is a significant factor in causing migraines.

Brain Bites and Guided Strategies

- Alcohol consumption is widely recognised for its ability to induce tension headaches and hangovers. Studies have shown alcohol to be a headache trigger in both migraine and non-migraine subjects.

- Alcoholic beverages contain various substances that can influence migraines, including ethanol, acetaldehyde, histamine, tyramine, glutamate, and nitric oxide.

- Among the various substances found in alcoholic drinks, red wine is particularly known for its higher susceptibility to trigger migraines, largely due to its inclusion of tannins.

- Due to the complex interplay of these vasoactive molecules, it's important to consume alcoholic beverages with caution or avoid altogether.

3.12 A Delicious Dilemma: Coffee and Chocolate

I felt that coffee and chocolate deserved their own section in this book. They are both known for their many health benefits, not to mention their deliciousness, yet they can be a controversial food for many migraine sufferers. Coffee is my first go-to when I sense a possible migraine knocking at the door, and it continually surprises me with its effectiveness, particularly in alleviating early morning headaches. The natural compound responsible for this alleviation of headaches is caffeine, which has a direct effect on normalising cerebral blood vessel activity and reducing pain transmission.

Caffeine, an alkaloid compound from the methylxanthine family, offers an amazing variety of health benefits, including effects on vasomotor function. This means that caffeine can enhance blood flow by either dilating or constricting blood vessels. In the context of migraine pathology, caffeine plays a crucial role by inhibiting adenosine receptors, which typically promote cerebral vasodilation. By blocking these receptors, caffeine reduces the release of inflammatory and pain agents that are normally triggered through the adenosine signalling pathway. If you would like to know more on the adenosine signalling pathway, turn to Section 2.8 in Chapter 2.

Caffeine is widely recognised as an analgesic and can improve the effectiveness in pain relief by 40% when combined with an anti-inflammatory drug.[98] There are some migraine drugs that contain added caffeine including the non-synthetic migraine medication ergotamine, which available in doses of 1 or 2 mg, combined with 100 mg of caffeine (refer to Chapter 1, Section 1.9 for further information on ergotamine). Caffeine is best administered during the vasoconstrictive phase of a migraine. In other words, early intervention will not only yield better results but also provide early relief. You can refer to Chapter 4, Section 4.6 for further insight into the vasoconstrictive phase of migraines.

It is worthy to note that some individuals, particularly those who regularly consume high amounts of coffee, abstaining from caffeine can trigger headaches or migraines. These caffeine withdrawal symptoms may be due to the upregulation of adenosine receptors in habitual coffee drinkers, leading to increased sensitivity to the uninhibited adenosine activity that occurs during caffeine abstinence. However, regular moderate coffee consumption can be highly beneficial for individuals susceptible to headaches and migraine.

Chocolate is also worthy for discussion because it is a topic of controversy and a mixed bag of information regarding migraines. There is also much misinformation found on the internet about cacao, and chocolate, and its active compounds.

Some evidence suggests that cacao or dark chocolate may benefit migraine sufferers, while there is also a lot of anecdotal evidence suggesting that cacao can trigger migraines. Similar to other migraine trigger foods, chocolate shows inconsistent outcomes in research settings. The variability of these outcomes depends on individual sensitivity to the chocolate trigger and the quantity consumed. Additionally, these triggers often synergistically contribute to a cumulative effect with other triggers, a phenomenon I term as the 'snowball effect'. These variables lead to an inconsistent association with chocolate and migraine, and reinforces the complexity of migraine triggers. If you would like to know more about the snowball effect of migraine triggers, turn to Section 2.5, in Chapter 2.

The variable nature of cacao as a migraine trigger prompted me to investigate the composition and processing of cocoa and chocolate, and I found some compelling evidence. Firstly, cacao, the raw product of chocolate, is the dried and fermented fruit of the Theobroma cacao tree.

The term 'fermented' might have caught your attention, and rightly so. If you have read Sections 3.2 and 3.8 about amines and glutamate in Chapter 3, you will understand the potential consequences of the fermentation process of certain foods.

Nevertheless, cacao in the form of dark chocolate is known to offer numerous health benefits, particularly rich in nutrients that can benefit migraine sufferers, including zinc, magnesium, selenium, and a range of flavanols which are responsible for most of the chocolate's health benefits due to their potent antioxidant activity.

This also includes serotonin, which is often touted as a beneficial compound present in chocolate. However, serotonin undergoes chemical decomposition during the long fermentation process of cocoa beans and eventually much of it disappears.[99]

The main ingredient in cacao that receives significant attention is theobromine, which is structurally similar to caffeine but is generally considered to be less stimulating. While cacao does contain small amounts of caffeine, theobromine is in higher abundance in comparison to caffeine, with a ratio of approximately 5:1.[100]

It is highly probable that the physiological effects of theobromine contribute to migraines. Medically, theobromine is used as a vasodilator for respiratory conditions such as asthma. Additionally, there is a suggestion that the theobromine found in chocolate may have beneficial effects on blood pressure[101] Furthermore, there is evidence indicating that theobromine can cross the blood-brain barrier, potentially leading to direct vasodilation of cerebral blood vessels[100]

Another migraine trigger found naturally high in cacao is glutamate. Due to the fermentation process, it can easily contain up to 3 gm of free glutamate per 100 gm of cacao. When choosing dark chocolate, the glutamate levels vary based on the cacao content. For example, dark chocolate with 50% cacao content may contain around 1.5 grams of glutamate per 100 grams, compared to dark chocolate with 90% cacao content, which can contain up to 3 grams of glutamate per 100 grams. Therefore, selecting dark chocolate with higher cacao content can significantly increase the levels of glutamate, potentially affecting migraine susceptibility. Glutamate and theobromine— the perfect storm for a migraine in waiting.

If you believe milk chocolate is safer because it contains less cacao mass, it's important to read the labels. You will find that chocolate manufacturers add extra glutamate, especially to milk chocolate, to enhance its chocolaty taste 'umami'. Check the ingredients list for 'flavouring,' which is another term for glutamate. The good news is, there are chocolate sources available without added glutamate, especially if you choose organic chocolate.

The other three migraine triggers present in chocolate are tyramine, phenylethylamine and polyphenols. Tyramine's trigger mechanism was discussed in this chapter in Section 3.5 via its vasoconstrictive effect and the activation of the stress hormone norepinephrine, which can further augment vasoconstriction. Phenylethylamine, on the other hand, has little evidence as a migraine trigger compared to other amines.

However, it is noteworthy that phenylethylamine can also release the stress hormone norepinephrine and affect changes in cerebral blood flow.[100] It may well be that these two physiological actions exert a cumulative effect with other migraine triggers.

Another notable aspect of phenylethylamine is its relatively high levels in cacao. Unlike serotonin, which breaks down and disappears during the fermentation process of the cacao bean, phenylethylamine actually increases in concentration.[99]

Another significant compound that can affect cerebral blood vessels are the polyphenols. These are a group of naturally occurring chemicals found in plant-based foods and are the holy grail of antioxidant activity. Polyphenols are found in unusually high quantities in cacao; in fact, 10% of dried cacao consists of polyphenols, with catechins, anthocyanins and proanthocyanidins as the most abundant flavonoids[102]

Polyphenols can cross the blood-brain barrier with great efficiency,[100] a fact I find truly compelling. The blood brain barrier evolved over millions of years to protect the brain from harmful substances while allowing only the most essential compounds to pass. The fact that 'polyphenols can pass with great efficiency' explains their profound protective benefits for brain tissue. These powerful antioxidants are recognized by our very biology as vital defenders of cognitive health, reinforcing the brain's resilience against oxidative stress and degeneration.

From a migraine perspective, polyphenols increase cerebral blood flow and enhance the production of the potent vasodilator nitric oxide (NO)[100] which plays a significant role in migraine pathogenesis. If you would like to know more on the role of NO, turn to Section 3.11 in this chapter.

Although chocolate's role as a migraine trigger is inconsistent, the presence of a wide variety of migraine-triggering compounds in cacao offers compelling insights into its potential effects. To delve deeper, I decided to conduct a chocolate-eating experiment, fully aware of the potential for adverse outcomes. Nevertheless, as researchers, we sometimes need to put ourselves on the line to test research theories.

From a pure chocolate perspective, my love for dark chocolate is exceptional, and I know from experience that consuming it does not consistently trigger a migraine. However, I began my experiment with a small amount, just 5 grams of 70-80% dark chocolate, and experienced no adverse effects. By my fourth experiment, I found dark chocolate to be highly effective in ameliorating tension headaches (constricted blood vessels). With this success, I decided to consume 5 grams of 80% dark chocolate during a mild migraine headache. Unfortunately, it had a dire outcome, accelerating and intensifying my migraine symptoms, a memorable experience I do not wish to revisit. In this experiment, I believe that my mild headache was already in the vasodilatory stage (migraine headache), and the chocolate enhanced this process.

Unlike coffee, using cocoa or dark chocolate to reduce headaches is a bit like playing Russian roulette because it is difficult to define where the vasoconstriction ends and vasodilation begins during a migraine event. Two experiments with 20 grams of 80% dark chocolate also led to a migraine. Conducting these experiments away from any other possible triggers suggests that, in my case, it depended on the quantity of chocolate and any pre-susceptibility with other triggers at play.

Brain Bites and Guided Strategies

Coffee and Caffeine:

1. Caffeine works by normalising cerebral blood vessel activity and reducing pain transmission and is best used in the early phase of a migraine for better results. For a speedy result with coffee, I recommend a short black. By adding a bit of sugar and milk will enhance the absorption of the caffeine and you should feel the benefit within 5-10 minutes. This can be taken with or without your usual migraine medication.

2. Regular, moderate coffee consumption can be beneficial for individuals susceptible to headaches and migraines and can be effective in alleviating early morning headaches and migraines. It is also good to be aware that abstaining from caffeine can trigger headaches in some habitual coffee drinkers.

Cocoa and Chocolate:

1. Cocoa and especially dark chocolate, contains compounds like theobromine, tyramine, phenylethylamine, glutamate and polyphenols. The effects of chocolate as a migraine trigger can vary depending on individual sensitivity, quantity consumed and other triggers present (the 'snowball effect'). Avoid added glutamate in commercial chocolate, labelled as flavouring.

2. It is important to note that individual responses to coffee and chocolate can vary, so what works for one person may not work for another. Keeping a migraine diary can help track triggers and responses to different foods and beverages, including coffee and chocolate, to better manage migraines.

3.13 Citric Acid

The first time I realised that citric acid could be a trigger for some individuals was while using certain nutritional supplements. Citric acid is commonly included in various supplements due to its function as a natural preservative. It has a tangy flavour, acts as a flavour enhancer, and specifically aids in mineral absorption.

I regularly recommended mineral supplements containing citrate specifically due to its efficiency in mineral absorption. However, infrequently, one of my patients would report that these supplements triggered migraines. Initially, this was perplexing, as I was confident that the minerals themselves were not to blame. My focus turned to the excipient. By simply switching the supplement, such as the form of magnesium citrate, to magnesium glycinate, I was able to provided immediate relief for that individual.

Excess citric acid itself is unlikely to directly cause an overproduction of glutamate in the body, though there are a few indirect mechanisms to consider, particularly for sensitive individuals.

In theory, an excess of citric acid could lead to increased levels of alpha-ketoglutarate, which is a precursor to glutamate. Although the body tightly regulates glutamate production based on its metabolic needs, excess glutamate production should not occur simply due to increased citric acid levels.

However, individuals with glutamate dysregulation, such as those with certain neurological conditions like migraines, may be more sensitive to changes in glutamate levels. Even slight increases in glutamate could potentially trigger a migraine event. The main culprit is most likely the activity of citric acid on the TRPV1 receptor, which directly stimulates pain pathways by promoting the release of pro-inflammatory neuropeptides like CGRP.

There are both natural and processed foods that contain citric acid. A good rule of thumb is that any sour food has the potential to contain citric acid. In natural foods, the sour taste typically comes from a combination of ascorbic acid (vitamin C) and citric acid, with many containing only minimal amounts of citric acid. Exceptions to this include citrus fruits like lemons, limes and oranges, where citric acid is present in large amounts. Other specific fruits, such as tomatoes and sour berries, also contain notable levels of citric acid.

In manufactured foods, checking the ingredient list is crucial, as many products contain citric acid. This ingredient is often used as a preservative or to provide a sour taste that enhances the flavour of the product.

When looking for citric acid on food labels, it is typically presented simply as 'citric acid', especially in processed foods, canned goods, beverages, and candies. You will find this ingredient is usually listed near the middle or end of the ingredients list. Citric acid may also be categorised under 'acidity regulator' or 'preservative (E330)'.

Below is a list of some common foods and beverages that contain citric acid:

Beverages

- Soft drinks, fruit juices and energy drinks.

Dairy Products

- Yoghurts – especially fruit-flavoured varieties.

Snacks and Confectionery

- Candy – especially sour candies, gummies and fruit-flavoured sweets.

- Baked goods – some cookies and cakes, granola and dried fruit bars.

Sauces and Condiments

- Ketchup, salad dressings (common in vinaigrettes and flavoured dressings) and mayonnaise.

Canned and Jarred Foods

- Canned vegetables, pickles, jams, and jellies.

Frozen Foods

- Frozen fruits and meals, and ice-creams.

Prepared and Processed Foods

- Instant noodles – often found in flavour packets.

- Meat products – such as some sausages and deli meats.

CHAPTER 4

Reducing the Sensitivity Factor

4.1 The Stress Profile

Stress serves as the primary driving force in the migraine process and exerts a significant influence on other triggers. The multidimensional effects of stress make it such that each one of us possesses a unique stress profile that can affect physical, emotional and mental wellbeing.

Stressors are dynamic and can vary in nature for each person and for each situation. Common personal stressors are deadlines, personal challenges, financial concerns, relationship issues, health problems, and major life changes.

Additionally, everyday hassles such as being late for work, experiencing traffic jams, facing long queues, or misplacing items can also contribute to stress. Unmistakably, there is a plethora of stressors that each and every one of us encounters, often without even being aware of their presence. Stressors accumulate over time, exacerbating our overall stress levels and eventually affecting our mental wellbeing.

Understanding someone's stress profile involves assessing both the specific stressors they encounter and their individual responses to those stressors. Factors such as coping mechanisms, resilience and the overall impact on their daily life contribute to the complexity of a stress profile. Additionally, a stress profile can be dynamic, changing over time as individuals experience different life events, adapt to new circumstances, or implement coping strategies. Recognising and analysing your stress profile can be valuable for tailoring interventions, providing support and developing strategies to manage stress effectively.

Let's face it, we all experience stress. Both psychological (mental) and physical stress are a natural part of the human experience. First and foremost, it's important to recognise that there is both good stress and bad stress. Occasional stress can be beneficial, as it builds bodily resilience, aids in coping, boosts confidence, and enhances performance during challenging times.

However, stress becomes detrimental when these moments become frequent or chronic and eventually break the body's resilience. Chronic stress will leave the body with persistent inflammation and adversely impact brain function. When bad stress is ignored, it can become the primary driver for migraines and a myriad of other health problems.

To successfully manage your stressors, it is crucial to have a good understanding of both mental and physical stressors. This includes understanding why they occur, how they occur, and how they can impact the frequency and severity of migraines in the long term. In the following pages, I will explain in depth the nature of stress from an evolutionary perspective and how it impacts the body in today's fast-paced world.

4.2 Mental Stress

Mental stress is a psychological response to how we perceive our environment. It often arises from situations or tasks we believe we cannot effectively cope with. This perceived stress triggers a biological process in the body known as the stress response.

The stress response is a primordial survival mechanism which allows the body to quickly react to any life-threatening situation. This activates the fear-defence system, often called the 'fight or flight system', as it readies the body for intense physical activity in response to a perceived threat. Once the danger has passed, the stress subsides, and the body returns to its normal state of balance. This is known as homeostasis.

Today, our stressors may differ from those of our prehistoric ancestors, but our biological coping mechanisms remain unchanged. Whether being chased by a tiger or simply running late for work and anticipating a stern boss, the chemical process of the stress response is the same.

*The key difference with modern stressors is that they are often psychological rather than real, immediate danger. They are conjured up in the mind—triggered by worries, social pressures and uncertainties, yet they still provoke the same stress response.

Essentially, the nervous system with which we evolved was not designed to deal with the daily grind of modern life. Any psychological and physical demands on the nervous system were meant to be brief and this encompassed the basic essential needs of hunting and food gathering, staying safe from any threats, keeping warm, and generally having little expectation for what is to come.

Today, our nervous system is in a perpetual state of activation. We find ourselves stressing about a myriad of things, trying to keep our lives neatly boxed into organised chaos as we juggle everyday tasks, demands, obligations, deadlines, and expectations. Mentally, we live a hectic life and therefore the psychological, emotional and physical stressors are a common challenge of modern life.

The external manifestation of mental stressors is emotional symptoms. When we feel overwhelmed and vulnerable, emotions can present as worry, apprehension, anxiety, and fear. When mental stress manifests into frustration or irritation, it can escalate into outbursts of anger or rage. While these emotions are a normal part of life, the frequent or chronic experiences of stress can lead to more serious health problems. Some of these tell-tale symptoms include:

- Anxiety
- Panic attacks
- Depression
- Despondency
- Poor sleep or insomnia

- Vivid dreams and nightmares
- Waking unrefreshed
- Poor appetite
- Headaches and migraines
- Aches and pains
- Fatigue
- High blood pressure
- Weight gain
- Muscle tension
- Jaw clenching and teeth grinding, predominantly at night
- Digestive problems
- Low libido

The stress response is primarily driven by the sympathetic nervous system and the immune system. When triggered, these systems release stress hormones like adrenaline and noradrenaline, which increase blood flow, heart rate and breathing to provide the muscles and brain with more glucose and oxygen. If stress persists, cortisol is released to further enhance the fight-or-flight response, aiming to restore homeostasis more quickly. However, cortisol also inhibits non-essential bodily functions during stress, such as digestion, hormone and insulin production, as well as general tissue repair.

The immune system also plays a role in stress, acting as a defence mechanism in case of injury and regulating the release of additional stress hormones and neurotransmitters that affect cognition and behaviour.[103] However, when these restorative systems are constantly activated due to frequent and chronic stress, homeostasis is not achieved. This prolonged activation leads to persistent inflammation, tissue damage and eventually, disease.

Stress affects us all differently, and it can contribute to various health issues over time. Naturopathic philosophy recognises that as individuals we all have inherent weaknesses and thus an increased susceptibility in certain body systems. Digestive function is particularly vulnerable to mental stress, often manifesting in symptoms of indigestion, poor appetite, heartburn, reflux, ulcers, and other related complaints. Stress can also lead to conditions such as high blood pressure or blood sugar imbalances. Additionally, the female reproductive system is sensitive to stress, potentially resulting in menstrual pain or menstrual irregularities.

Inherent weaknesses can refer to various aspects where individuals may be more susceptible to certain health issues or conditions due to genetic factors, physiological characteristics or environmental influences. These inherent weaknesses are not necessarily debilitating or insurmountable but will require individuals to take extra focus to engage in specific health practices to manage or mitigate their effects. For migraine sufferers, this scenario is all too familiar as their nervous system harbors this inherent vulnerability.

4.3 Physical Stress

As noted earlier in this chapter, stress can impact not only our mental but also our physical wellbeing, serving as a significant trigger for migraineurs.

During a mental stress response, muscles naturally tense up as a reflex to guard against potential injury and pain. This tension helps protect the body during times of heightened alertness. Once the stress subsides, muscle tension typically diminishes, and the body returns to a state of homeostasis.

Chronic stress often leads to persistent muscle tension, particularly in the shoulders and neck. This ongoing tension can lead to fatigue, muscle spasms and pain. Prolonged muscle tension can subsequently trigger an immune response and activate the trigeminovascular system, which is involved in the development of migraines. Other physical stressors that can contribute to this tension include electrolyte imbalances, such as sodium and magnesium depletion, as well as dehydration.

Another prevalent trigger of physical stress is the physical condition of our muscles, if they are either weak or overexerted. This topic is further explained in Chapter 2, Section 2.4, 'Identifying your triggers'. From a physical perspective, stress often manifests through poor posture, which can be exacerbated by weak muscle integrity and a lack of physical activity. An individual's ability to cope with physical stress is closely tied to their level of physical fitness. Therefore, maintaining good muscle integrity requires regular physical activity.

From a physiological perspective, physical activity reaches way beyond merely promoting good muscle tone and muscle integrity. Muscle movement helps to remove daily metabolic waste products via the lymphatic system and ushers them to the excretory organs via liver and kidneys. This task is crucial for reducing free radicals and maintaining homeostasis. Healthy, active muscles not only oversee immune and neuroendocrine functions but they also regulate blood glucose levels and release endorphins, imparting a sense of energy and contentment that ultimately leads to reduced stress.

Regardless of whether your challenges entail mental or physical stress, it is crucial to understand that you alone have the ultimate power to effectively address them. Self-help empowers you to take control of your mental and emotional wellbeing. With this approach, you can choose from various practices and techniques that can effectively help you to manage stress levels and promote overall mental health. These may include mindfulness meditation, deep breathing exercises, journaling, regular physical activities, engaging in hobbies, seeking social support, and setting personal boundaries to manage stressors effectively. By recognising the effectiveness of self-help, you can proactively address stress in your life and cultivate resilience to navigate challenges more effectively.

Brain Bites and Guided Strategies

- Understanding the impact of mental and physical stress is crucial for effectively managing your wellbeing. While your body's stress response mechanisms have evolved to handle immediate short-term threats, chronic stressors can lead to both physical and mental health issues.

- To address these challenges, it's important to adopt proactive strategies. Daily self-help practices will help to calm the nervous system, strengthen the coping mechanism, and adapt the mind to be less reactive. For further insights into the effects of stress on your health and wellbeing, I highly recommend you read the following sections: 4.4 'Stress Adaptation', and 4.5 'Feed your Stress'.

1. In The Therapy Kit, you will find the following self-help strategies and treatments. Refer to 'Stress Relief Strategies' in Section 5.8, including Subsections 5.8.1 through to 5.8.4.

4.4 Stress Adaptation: A Matter of Brain Plasticity

The brain is a dynamic and adaptive organ, capable of changing its structure and function in response to the environment. This ability, known as brain plasticity or neuroplasticity, is particularly evident in the context of migraines. The migraine-prone brain is a compelling example of this adaptability, as it becomes more sensitive to stressors and altered levels of regulatory neurotransmitters and hormones. Neuroplasticity involves the brain's capacity to reorganise itself by forming new neural connections. This adaptive response is a key mechanism that enables the organism to adapt, survive and potentially thrive in a changing environment.

Adaptation of brain plasticity can be beneficial or harmful depending on the type of stimuli the brain interprets. Typically, brain plasticity is crucial during growth, learning, memory formation, and cognitive behaviours, a process of brain adaptation that is continuous throughout an individual's life. What has also been shown to affect brain plasticity are brain disorders, and migraine is one such disorder that alters the structure and function in certain brain regions.

Two factors that have a direct impact on brain plasticity and alter the structure and function in certain brain regions are stress and inflammation, both of which are prominent in more chronic migraine disorder.[104] When stress becomes chronic, it can result in prolonged neuroinflammation, which may negatively affect brain function and increase the risk of various neurological and degenerative disorders.[105]

The three key regions of the brain involved in how we react to, and cope with stress are the amygdala, hippocampus and prefrontal cortex.

The amygdala is responsible for detecting and responding to potential threats. It plays a crucial role in the processing of emotions, particularly fear and aggression. When the amygdala perceives a threat, it can trigger the 'fight or flight' response, preparing the body to deal with the perceived danger.

In contrast, the hippocampus is involved in processing the stressful experience after the initial response. It helps with thinking and understanding, as well as regulating emotions and actions. The hippocampus is also crucial for learning and memory, particularly in forming new memories and integrating them into existing knowledge. In other words, the ability of the hippocampus allows it to process the stressful experience to help the individual understand, learn from, and potentially cope with, subsequent stressors in the future.

The amygdala and hippocampus relay this information to the prefrontal cortex, which plays a crucial role in regulating emotional responses and decision-making during stressful situations.

Over time, the frequent and chronic bombardment of stress can adversely impact brain plasticity, leading to structural changes in these brain regions. These changes can result in an enhanced responsiveness and sensitivity to stress stimuli.

The adaptive plasticity from ongoing stress increases the size of the amygdala to help strengthen the response to subsequent stressors and makes it more sensitised and responsive to perceived stress. These changes eventually lead to more robust and prolonged stress reactions.[106,107]

In contrast, the prefrontal cortex and the hippocampus shrink and can lead to impaired concentration and memory.[106,107] This stress adaptation can be characterised by more frequent or chronic anxiety, depressive thoughts, irritability, and short-temperedness.

'Frequent and chronic stress will structurally remodel and adapt various brain regions to be more responsive and prone to subsequent stressors.'

While many migraines typically occur sporadically and acutely, I belief that an increase in migraine frequency and chronic migraine may also be associated with underlying neuroinflammation. Chronic inflammation triggers oxidative stress, which involves the accumulation of harmful by-products from cellular and immune processes, further impacting inflammation. These processes can significantly impact brain function and structure, resulting in cellular damage and disruptions in neuronal connections. Consequently, this leads to neurotransmitter dysregulation and increases the likelihood of mood disorders like depression, chronic anxiety and cognitive decline.[108,109]

According to two studies, the most frequently observed results in migraine-affected brains include changes in volume of white and grey brain matter, as well as indications of small ischemic stroke-like lesion.[110,111] These lesions are commonly referred to as white matter lesions, which are a marker of small blood vessel disease. However, with further research, I found that these brain structure anomalies are also common in non-migraineur subjects,[112] which means that the lesions are not clinically specific to the migraine brain.

Nevertheless, it is important to note that these are irregularities that are believed to be the cause of infections, metabolic disorders like cardiovascular disease, diabetes, and degenerative changes,[112] in which inflammation and oxidative stress are the underlying drivers.

In conclusion, ongoing stress can lead to structural changes in the brain, which affect how we perceive and respond to stressors. These changes can contribute to the frequency and the chronicity of migraines.

Brain Bites and Guided Strategies

- The brain's ability to change and adapt its structure and function in response to the environment is known as brain plasticity or neuroplasticity. This process is crucial for adaptation to the environment.

- Chronic stressors and consequent adaptation of brain plasticity can make the brain more responsive and prone to subsequent stressors.

- Understanding the role of brain plasticity in migraines highlights the importance of managing stress and inflammation and oxidative stress.

- Restoring brain plasticity relies on a holistic approach with a combination of lifestyle and dietary modifications. For the most effective and personalised intervention, I strongly advise you to consult with a naturopathic clinician. Their expertise can ensure optimal results by tailoring the intervention to your specific needs and health profile.

The following protocols are a framework that helps to restore brain plasticity. These can be found in The Therapy Kit, Chapter 5.

1. Stress reduction: managing mental and physical stress through practices such as meditation, mindfulness and 'me' time. For a comprehensive guide on managing stress, refer to Section 5.8.

2. Immune regulation: For addressing underlying inflammation and modulating immune response, refer to Section 5.12.

3. Sleep is critical for brain plasticity, including the formation of new neural connections in response to learning, experience and damaged neurons. It also supports overall brain flexibility and adaptability. For more insights into the benefits of good sleep, refer to Subsection 5.8.4.

4. Nutrition to address oxidative stress: An enriching diet in high nutrient dense foods to enhance the body's nutrient pools in healthy fats, antioxidants, quality protein, and essential vitamins and minerals. To help maintain optimal antioxidant capacity, refer to Subsection 5.10.1.

5. Consult your naturopathic clinician to help with a personalised dietary protocol.

6. Exercise: Regular physical activity has been shown to promote brain plasticity and improve cognitive function. Refer to Section 5.8.2 for more information.

4.5 Feed your Stress: Improving Bodily Resilience

Stress is an innate part of the body's survival, and it is not something that we can switch off. As you are now aware, there exists both good and bad stress, and to maintain a healthy, balanced stress response, you must address your stress profile through two key approaches.

Firstly, you need to reduce your stressors with anti-stress techniques, and secondly, you need to feed your stress response. A healthy stress response needs to be nurtured by ensuring the body has access to the necessary nutrients for its crucial metabolic response. The body has an incredible ability to adapt and maintain homeostasis, but for optimal function, it requires an adequate supply of nutrients.

However, nutrient status is mostly an overlooked area in mental health. Stress significantly impacts nutrient levels by increasing nutrient utilisation and impairing digestive absorption. Chronic or frequent stress will deplete nutrient reserves as the body's heightened demand may not be met due to compromised digestion. This depletion not only affects the efficiency of the stress response but also has significant implications for other crucial metabolic pathways, particularly those involved in neurotransmitter and hormone synthesis, immune regulation and reducing oxidative stress. These pathways play a vital role in influencing mood, cognition and immune response.

Insufficient dietary intake and compromised digestive function can worsen the depletion of nutrient reserves. Consequently, resources will be redirected away from producing neurotransmitters essential for a positive mood. Instead, the body prioritises supporting the stress response as the primary goal of the fight-or-flight system to ensure survival. This redirection of nutrients can contribute to the development of anxiety and depression in individuals experiencing frequent or chronic stress.

Interestingly, the synthesis of primary stress hormones like adrenaline, noradrenaline and cortisol uses the same precursor nutrients needed for the synthesis of positive mood neurotransmitters such as serotonin and GABA. These nutrients include Vitamins B5, B3, B5, B6, B9, and Vitamin C, as well as minerals like magnesium and zinc.

Therefore, prioritising the production of stress hormones will deplete the availability of these nutrients needed for the synthesis of good mood neurotransmitters.

This highlights the importance of maintaining sufficient nutrient intake to support both stress management and mood stability.

In a state of inadequate nutrient supply, the stress
response will shunt nutrients
away from the production of good-mood neurotransmitters.

When nutrient deficiencies persist and there is a diminished delivery of nutrients for good-mood neurotransmitter production, the psychological resilience of the mental and emotional coping mechanism begins to fail, and a plethora of health problems arise. Common symptoms include heart palpitations, and mood changes, which develop into anxiety and depression. Often there is a shift in body weight and poor sleep, which can lead to insomnia and fatigue, and the beginnings of aches and pains in muscles and joints. The shift in mood can affect appetite and digestive problems, which will further impact nutrient pools and perpetuate the cycle of stress, inflammation and oxidative stress.

Brain Bites and Guided Strategies

- There are both good and bad types of stress and maintaining a healthy stress response involves reducing stressors and ensuring the body has access to an optimal nutrient supply.

- Chronic stress can deplete essential nutrient reserves, affecting metabolic pathways crucial for mood, cognition and immune response.

- Chronic stress and inadequate nutrient intake can contribute to inflammation and oxidative stress, which in turn can exacerbate the effects of stress on the body.

The following treatment options can be found in The Therapy Kit, Chapter 5.

1. Addressing stress: Stress can deplete nutrients, increase inflammation and elevate oxidative stress. For more information, refer to 'Stress Relief Strategies' in Section 5.8 and its subsections, including 'Feed Your Stress' in Subsection 5.8.3.

2. Quality Sleep: Sleep helps regulate the production of stress hormones like cortisol. When sleep -deprived, the body's cortisol levels can remain elevated, leading to heightened stress. Sufficient sleep ensures that cortisol levels are regulated, reducing stress.

3. Chronic sleep deprivation: Poor sleep is linked to mental health disorders such as anxiety and depression, which can increase stress levels. Refer to 'The Power of Quality Sleep' in Subsection 5.8.4.

4.6 Serotonin in Rebound Vasodilation: The Premise from Headache to Migraine

Before delving into the intricate role of serotonin in migraine pathology, it is crucial to understand that the alleviation of migraines primarily depends on restoring cerebral vascular equilibrium with serotonin playing a central role in this complex process. Serotonin activity is dynamic with levels fluctuating in response to various external and internal factors such as mood, stress, diet, and exposure to light. Moreover, serotonin receptors exhibit the ability to upregulate or downregulate in response to changes in serotonin levels. It is this dynamic nature of serotonin that creates susceptible periods for individuals prone to migraines.

In this section, we will explore how serotonin is involved in migraine pathology and how maintaining optimal serotonin levels can help prevent migraines.

Serotonin is involved in a wide range of physiological and behavioural functions, notably in modulating vascular tone and central capillary blood flow. Supported by the immune and neuroendocrine systems, serotonin helps maintain a dynamic equilibrium in vascular tone and blood flow, adapting them to physiological and biochemical challenges to stabilise internal conditions.

The significance of serotonin's functions is highlighted by its production in various tissues, particularly in the brain and gastrointestinal tract. Serotonin serves as a crucial mediator in the complex interplay among the nervous, immune and cardiovascular systems.

In the context of vascular tone and blood flow regulation, serotonin acts on specialised receptors located on smooth muscle cells lining blood vessels. When released, serotonin can induce changes in vascular tone by narrowing or widening of blood vessels. This ability to modulate vascular tone is vital for maintaining optimal blood pressure, ensuring adequate blood flow, and oxygenation, especially critical in brain tissue.

While other excitatory neurotransmitters such as noradrenaline, glutamate and dopamine actively participate in the migraine process, it is serotonin that holds a paramount position in regulating the activity of these excitatory neurotransmitters and overall neurological balance. This means that serotonin activity has the capacity to maintain regulatory order of cerebral blood vessels and the trigeminovascular system. Effectively, optimal serotonin activity inhibits neurogenic inflammation and pain.

However, when serotonin activity is suboptimal, these pathways are unopposed, releasing the potent vasodilatory and inflammatory compounds, including adenosine, nitric oxide (NO) and calcitonin gene-related peptide (CGRP), which have shown to be greatly elevated during the headache phase of a migraine event.[71]

There is a divergence of opinions within the research field regarding serotonin levels in individuals with migraines. Some studies have suggested that there may be an association between elevated serotonin levels and migraines, while other research propose a link between decreased serotonin availability or dysfunction of serotonin. Although the relationship between serotonin levels and migraines is complex and not fully understood, it is important to point out that both viewpoints are correct, as serotonin levels will fluctuate throughout the various phases of the migraine event. Research in the field of migraines is inherently complex and often yields conflicting findings. The heterogeneity of migraine as a condition poses significant challenges in drawing definitive conclusions and ongoing difficulty in establishing consistent results.

Returning to the topic of serotonin status, it is important to note that over 90% of serotonin is produced in the digestive system, and operates independently from brain serotonin, given its inability to cross the blood-brain barrier.[113] Nevertheless, growing evidence suggests that intestinal bacteria possess the ability to influence the expression of brain serotonin and other neurotransmitters, along with their precursors and receptors. This communication is thought to involve blood and vagus nerve pathways, collectively referred to as the gut-brain axis.[113] However, the precise mechanisms of this biochemical process remain unclear.[113,114] Furthermore, it is important to note that serotonin is stored in platelets and platelets, which have the ability to cross the blood-brain barrier.[115] It therefore could be postulated that brain tissue has an available source of serotonin from the peripheral circulation.

There are many factors that influence serotonin activity, including nutrient deficiencies that can impact the production of serotonin, its receptors or its transporters. Daily sunlight exposure is necessary for effective serotonin synthesis. Conditions such as depression, anxiety, bipolar disorder, and schizophrenia are associated with suboptimal serotonin levels and can directly impact serotonin activity in the brain.[116] Additionally, the nervous system, influenced by mental and physiological stressors, plays a significant role in adversely affecting serotonin activity.

The steroid cortisol, a stress-induced hormone, has a direct effect in diminishing serotonin levels. It does this by promoting the uptake of serotonin by lymphocytes and platelets, consequently removing it from circulation. This intricate relationship between cortisol and serotonin involves not only removal from circulation but also influences the synthesis and release of serotonin.[117] Studies have shown a correlation between elevated cortisol levels and diminished serotonin activity, particularly in conditions such as episodic migraines. In chronic migraines, the association is even more pronounced, highlighting the significance of stress in serotonin regulation.[118]

Cortisol can also influence the synthesis of serotonin through the availability of its precursor, the essential amino acid, tryptophan, which serves as the building block for serotonin. Cortisol does this by increasing the activity of an enzyme called tryptophan dioxygenase, which diverts tryptophan away from serotonin synthesis and leads to a decrease in serotonin production.[119]

For migraineurs, the fluctuations in serotonin levels can have a more pronounced effect because of their nervous system's heightened sensitivity. According to Panconesi, who undertook a revision of studies in assessing the changes of serotonin parameters in migraine patients, concluded that migraineurs tend to have lower levels of serotonin when compared to non-migraineurs. Furthermore, the assessment of serotonin reactivity in the hand vein to evaluate vasoconstrictive activity revealed greater sensitivity in migraineurs when compared to non-migraineurs. Additionally, females exhibited higher sensitivity than males.[93] This depicted sensitivity typically leads to an overreactive neurological and immune response on cerebral blood flow and consequential migraine symptoms.

The fluctuations in serotonin are a normal stress response, but for the migraineur this physiological scenario is greatly exaggerated. If we observe such a physiological event in individuals who do not experience migraines, we generally find that the exposure to a stress-inducing situation results in no symptoms or may result in a tension-type headache, triggered by a vasoconstrictive effect via sympathetic activity. As the stress diminishes, neurotransmitter levels normalise, facilitating the return of the body to a state of homeostasis.

In comparison, the hypersensitive state of the migraineur's nervous system brings about a more intensified and prolonged duration of the vasoconstrictive phase and reduced blood flow. As a result, the hypoperfusion, or suboptimal blood flow in cerebral tissue, initiates a coordinated immune response to restore normal blood flow, leading to an overcompensated, exaggerated inflammatory response. This hyperactivity manifests as a 'rebound vasodilation', which is a key component in the development of migraines.

In migraine research, there is a noticeable lack of discussion surrounding rebound vasodilation. This oversight likely stems from the limited emphasis on vasoconstriction and yet, it plays an integral part in the early stages of a migraine.

From a clinical and personal experience, I have learned that a migraine event, more often than not, begins with a vasoconstrictive headache. This can be anything from a tension headache, pain around the temples, at the base of the neck or skull, or a deep pain behind the eyes. The shift from constricted to dilated blood vessels is not recognised and the transition may occur slowly or quickly and is mostly likely dependent on the severity of the triggers and the chronicity of migraine.

There are some studies that support the theory of a vasoconstrictive phase prior to a vasodilatory phase. According to the authors, this was evident by an unusually diminished cerebral blood flow during the vasoconstrictive phase, followed by a heightened cerebral blood flow during the vasodilatory phase, with headache pain in both phases.[120-123] What is noteworthy, is one author's comment explaining an 'abnormal' cerebral blood flow in specific brain regions during both constrictive and dilatory phases, which may indicate that classic physiological sensitivity and hyperreactivity of blood vessel activity during the pathological event of a migraine.

While serotonin and noradrenaline primarily drive the vasoconstrictive phase another vasoconstrictor that directly stimulates the HPA axis and contributes to pain sensation is a small protein called endothelin-1 (ET1). Observed in a small number of studies, ET1 was found to be present in high plasma concentration in the early stages of migraine attacks.[124,125]

ET1 is a potent vasoconstrictor and generally known to express in situations of vascular damage with disease or trauma. More recent research has observed the expression of this protein during stress response, including anxiety and depression.[125,126]

Interestingly, there is evidence of ET1 expressed in a part of the brain region called the amygdala, which is the centre of emotional response and the home of neurotransmitters glutamate. In this region, ET1 is involved in the neuroendocrine stress response by activating the HPA axis, which directly affects anxiety, and the induction of a vasoconstrictive effect in preparation for the fight or flight system.[103] ET1 also can induces pain and sensitises other pain receptors. Notably, ET1 also stimulates and releases the vasodilatory migraine substances CGRP, nitric oxide and prostaglandin I2 (PGI2),[125] which suggests that ET1 may play an active part in rebound vasodilation.

Brain Bites and Guided Strategies

The shift in serotonin is not imperceptible and you will have ample time for some preventative measures. This will take a bit of practice, but you will experience subtle or quite notable changes in mood, which can occur between 12 – 42 hours prior to a migraine attack. You will find a list of these symptoms in the 'The premonition phase' in Chapter 2, Section 2.6.

- The primary factors causing serotonin levels to drop include stressors, chronic pain and nutritional deficiencies.

Outlined below are specific treatment solutions designed to help you achieve and maintain optimal serotonin levels, The following strategies are available in the Therapy Kit, Chapter 5.

- Physical Activity: Boost your serotonin production. Refer to Subsection 5.8.2.

- Sunlight: Natural light increases serotonin levels. You will find more information on this in Chapter 4, Section 4.10 'The Power of Sunlight'.

- A healthy diet: Up to 90% of serotonin is produced in the gut. Refer to Section 5.10 'Striving for Optimal Gut Function'.

- Strive for 'Happiness'. Cheerfulness boosts serotonin, and vice versa.

- Address stressors: Refer to 'Stress Relief Strategies' in Section 5.8 and Subsections 5.8.1, 5.8.2 and 5.8.4.

- Improve availability of cofactors for the serotonin pathway: Refer to 'Feed Your Stress' in Subsection 5.8.3.

For migraineurs, sleep is a vulnerable time where
underlying stress, shallow breathing and
hypoxia sets the stage for hypnic headaches and morning migraines.'

4.7 The Role of Hypoxia in the Pathology of Migraines

Hypoxia is the condition in which the body is deprived of adequate oxygen delivery to its tissues.

In the context of migraine, hypoxia refers to a potential decrease in oxygen levels in the brain, and that it can contribute to the activation of certain pathways in the brain that are involved in pain perception and the initiation of migraine attacks.

Several studies have validated that hypoxia can trigger or exacerbate migraines. It is known to occur in cortical spreading depression (CSD) and visual aura.[127,128] CSD is a phenomenon characterised by a wave of neuronal depolarisation followed by a period of suppressed neuronal activity, and it seems to be associated with migraine aura. Some people experience visual auras, which can range from a perception of flickering or flashing lights like fireworks, or shimmering, zigzagging lights that start off small and expand to the periphery of the visual field.

Others will experience blind spots or changes in the perception of colours. Studies commonly address visual auras as precursors to a migraine attack; however, it is noteworthy that these visual auras can manifest spontaneously and inexplicably, seemingly out of the blue and without a migraine headache—in other words, a silent migraine. Besides the presentation of visual aura in a silent migraine, other symptom presentations, which are highly individualised, can include nausea, dizziness and sensitivity to light and sounds.

Migraines known as high-altitude headache are also influenced by hypoxia. Researchers conduct these studies in high-altitude areas during mountain climbing expeditions where individuals are naturally exposed to lower oxygen levels. At high altitudes, the concentration of oxygen in the air decreases as air pressure drops. This decrease in oxygen availability leads to a hypoxia-induced cerebral vasodilation and a consequential migraine.[129] Interestingly, several epidemiological studies have reported a higher prevalence of migraine among populations residing at high altitudes, such as those in the mountain regions of the Himalayas and Andes, when compared to low lying regions.[130-132] Moreover, the migraine characteristics of these high-altitude populations are more frequent, more severe and longer in duration during migraine attacks.[131]

Another cause of suboptimal oxygen triggering migraine is individuals who have been diagnosed with a 'patent foramen ovale' (PFO). PFO is a congenital heart condition where a small opening persists between the right and left atria (upper chambers) of the heart after birth. It is estimated to be present in about 25% of the general population. This type of hypoxia occurs particularly when deoxygenated blood returns to the right atrium of the heart and mixes with oxygenated arterial blood in the left atrium.[133] These individuals have shown to benefit from supplemental oxygen.[134] It is important to note that not all individuals with PFO experience migraines, and secondly, intervention to close the hole in the atrial wall will reduce the frequency of migraines but not resolve them.[135] This suggests that there may be an underlying sensitivity to the migraine condition that is already present.

While hypoxia has been recognised as a potential migraine trigger, it is not widely acknowledged or discussed. Understandably, hypoxia typically manifests in severe circumstances and is not commonly observed in the broader migraine-affected demographic. Nonetheless, exploring the connection between hypoxia and migraines could offer valuable insights into the complex nature of migraine triggers. Potentially, the term 'pseudo-hypoxia' is particularly relevant given the hypersensitive and hyperexcitable neuronal processes, where even minor stimuli can provoke and amplify reactions in migraine susceptible individuals.

Pseudo-hypoxia refers to a condition where minor changes in oxygen levels do not indicate a true deficiency of oxygen. However, these minor alterations can significantly disrupt cellular processes in ways that mimic the effects of hypoxia and consequently increase the susceptibility of a migraine.

Subsequent ways in which pseudo-hypoxia can affect metabolic efficiency are firstly through peripheral vascular constriction via sympathetic activity (stress). This can lead to suboptimal blood flow in cerebral arteries, followed by the release of pain receptors (nociceptors) and the potent vasoactive substance adenosine and nitric oxide.[136] Adenosine, in particular, is released in response to low oxygen levels and acts as a potent vasodilator by orchestrating the release of glutamate and CGRP.[137]

Another mechanism that leads to pseudo-hypoxia is mitochondrial dysfunction. The mitochondria is the cell's generator and is responsible in the production of adenosine triphosphate (ATP), which is used as a source of chemical energy. A lack of oxygen impairs this energy production, resulting in a progressive hypoxic state that increases the production of reactive oxygen species (ROS), leading to oxidative stress. Oxidation can damage cells and tissues, contributing to inflammation and pain, both of which are key components of migraine pathology. Mitochondrial dysfunction can also be caused by the disruption of calcium homeostasis, which can lead to neuronal hyperexcitability, a condition often seen in migraine patients.[138]

Calcium influx into cells is suggested to play a role in causing cortical spreading depression. This process reduces cellular energy production, increases oxidative stress, and triggers the release of migraine-inducing compounds, all of which are efforts by the body to restore cellular order.

In this situation, once again, the body experiences a condition of pseudo-hypoxia, where it perceives that cells are not receiving enough oxygen. This perception leads to the widening of arteries to increase blood flow and oxygenation. Nitric oxide is the central player involved in this process.[138]

There is one more important factor that can lead to subclinical hypoxia, which we need to be aware of, and that is shallow breathing. Unbeknown to many, shallow breathing is a common phenomenon in the general population, not to mention the migraine community. Furthermore, susceptibility to subclinical hypoxia can increase during sleep, as muscles are in a more relaxed state and breathing patterns become quieter or subdued during the various sleep stages. For the migraineur, sleep is a vulnerable time when stress, shallow breathing and hypoxia set the stage for hypnic headaches and morning migraines.

4.8 Hypoxia in Sleep Disordered Breathing

Another obscure migraine trigger is nocturnal hypoxia. This is a state where there is insufficient oxygen in body tissue to maintain optimal physiological processes. A hypoxic state in the brain leads to a potent vasodilatory effect to improve cerebral circulation. This is triggered by a rise in carbon dioxide (hypercapnia) and activation of the sympathetic nervous system, resulting in the release of nitric oxide and other potent vasodilators.[139,140]

Hypoxia is not generally addressed in migraine sufferers, but should be considered, especially in individuals who regularly wake with a headache or migraine, and who may have a sleep disordered breathing condition.

Sleep disordered breathing (SDB) is often overlooked as a trigger for migraine. SDB is prevalent, and some studies suggest that up to 80% of people who suffer from this condition will be undiagnosed.[141]

SDB can present with various degrees of severity from a mild 'hypopnea', where the airway is narrow and partially obstructed, to an 'apnoea', where there is a temporary cessation of breathing due to a fully obstructed airway. When optimal breathing is disrupted, it adversely affects blood oxygen levels (hypoxia) and increases carbon dioxide in the body tissue.

It is well documented that the long-term counteractive effects on the body can lead to health issues, including high blood pressure, stroke, cardiovascular disease, and diabetes.[142] Individuals are also more likely to develop sleep deprivation, anxiety, depression, and fatigue, which can greatly affect the frequency and severity of headaches and migraines.[143]

Hypopnea is more common than we believe, and it often goes undetected by the sufferer as symptoms are less severe than when compared to apnoea. It presents as very short intervals of shallow breathing caused by partial obstruction and can affect between 30-90% of air flow, and reduce oxygen saturation from 3-6%.[144] Changes in oxygen saturation activate the sympathetic nervous system to reinstate order of the body's oxygen levels, which may result in vasomotor changes, activation of stress hormones and nocturnal waking and stretching to increase ventilation and blood flow.

What causes the partial or full obstruction of the airway is mostly the tongue. The oropharyngeal airway is located just behind the tongue and is only 8 mm in diameter for adults. During sleep, gravity and muscle relaxation cause the tongue to fall back and normally reduce the airway opening. However, the impact of ageing, alcohol consumption, and diminished elastic integrity of the muscle tissue around the airway, can impact air flow further during muscle relaxation.

Reduced elastic integrity is also evident for women progressing into menopause as the elasticity of muscle tissue diminishes with the drop in oestrogen and may therefore further impact SDB. This may cause the tongue to partially or fully obstruct the airway, causing the person to snore. Other less common factors of SDB include thyroid disease, enlarged tonsils and acid reflux.

Excess weight is a prominent aggravator for SDB. Fat deposits in the neck and throat region will further impact apnoea symptoms on the relaxed airway during sleep. The weight of excess abdominal fat can also add pressure on the chest and reduce lung volume. This can lead to shallow breathing and reduces vital tissue oxygenation.[142] According to a longitudinal study, that observed weight gain and changes in SDB, moderate weight loss can significantly influence the management of SDB.

On the flip side, a 10% weight gain is associated with a six-fold increase in the likelihood of developing moderate to severe SDB.[142]

Chronic SDB leads to physiological and psychological conditions due to sleep deprivation and suboptimal oxygen saturation, and can manifest into daytime sleepiness, depression and further weight gain.[145]

Another susceptibility to SDB is in the upper airway anatomy. A narrow palate and retro positioning of the lower jaw further increases the risk of a partial or full obstruction when muscle tissue is in a relaxed state during sleep.[146]

The retro position of the jaw is a condition called retrognathia and is characterised by the positioning of the lower jaw being posterior to the upper jaw. This results in the appearance of a pronounced overbite, where the lower teeth are situated noticeably behind the upper teeth. In a relaxed state of sleep the retrograde jaw falls back even further, obstructing the airway.

Children and adolescence who are susceptible to recurrent headaches need to be examined for SDB, especially if there is a recurrent swelling of the adenoids and tonsils from chronic infection.

The consequences of SDB on brain tissue and migraine susceptibility is the impact in the frequency and severity of both nocturnal headaches, morning headaches and migraines on rising. Early morning headaches can generally be eased with deep breathing or getting up and about. Keep in mind that these headaches can progress into a migraine, especially if other triggers are involved. It is the mild and inconspicuous hypopnea symptoms which are mostly overlooked or not recognised as SDB and yet, can have a profound impact for migraine and headache sufferers.

Here is a list of suggestive sleep-disordered breathing (SDB) symptoms that you can familiarise yourself with. I recommend educating your partner about these symptoms to enhance their understanding and provide valuable support.

- Habitual snoring or intermittent snoring
- Waking with a snort or gasping sounds
- Frequent waking
- Light sleep or disrupted sleep
- Waking with feeling of anxiety or panic
- Waking with a feeling of shortness of breath
- Partner telling you that you snore
- Nightmares or disturbing dreams

- Frequent mild headaches during the night and early mornings
- Early morning headache improved with deep breathing or rising
- Experiencing a great need to stretch your body during the night.
- Stretching can be intense or frequent.
- Feeling sleepy
- Lack of energy at rising

4.9 Shallow Breathing and the Stress Response

Understanding your breath and cultivating healthy breathing practices can significantly reduce the occurrence of migraines and headaches. Shallow breathing can result in subclinical hypoxia in cerebral tissue, triggering migraine episodes. Additionally, conditions like sleep-disordered breathing, including hypopnea and apnoea (as discussed in Section 4.8) can also lead to subclinical hypoxia. In this chapter, we delve deeper into the intricate relationship between shallow breathing and stress, emphasising its direct impact on migraines and headaches.

The prevalent habit of shallow breathing is a widespread occurrence in today's fast-paced and stress-ridden society. While it may seem inconspicuous, shallow breathing poses a significant health risk by directly engaging the body's stress response mechanism. This type of breathing is often linked to stress, anxiety and poor breathing habits. Moreover, factors such as a sedentary lifestyle and certain health conditions can contribute to the development of shallow breathing patterns. The suboptimal oxygen delivery will further contribute to the cycle of stress and anxiety because it limits the amount of oxygen reaching the body's tissues and can lead to feelings of breathlessness, increased tension, and tachycardia (rapid heartbeat).

Shallow breathing is not confined to daytime; it can occur during sleep, and can potentially be worsened by sleep itself. Breathing significantly decreases during all sleep stages compared to wakefulness, particularly during rapid-eye-movement (REM).[147] Considering these sleep-related changes in breathing patterns, combined with other triggers, such as bringing your stress to bed, sensitivity to certain foods or cyclic drops in estrogen levels, may increase the likelihood of early morning migraines.

From a clinical perspective, I have found that susceptibility to a migraine attack most commonly occurs in the early hours of the morning, between 2 am and 4 am. Sleep is a vulnerable time for the body, during which neurotransmitters like serotonin undergo a shift to a nocturnal function. The fluctuations in serotonin levels are not only associated with stress responses but also align with the natural circadian rhythm. Additionally, neurotransmitters such as norepinephrine, histamine and glutamate, which typically exhibit heightened activity during wakefulness, show reduced activity during the Rapid Eye Movement (REM) phase of sleep.[148]

Besides early morning migraines, you may also be experiencing early morning headaches. These are commonly referred to as hypnic headaches, often known as 'alarm clock' headaches, as they usually wake you at the same time during the night, generally around 2-4 am. Interestingly, hypnic headaches tend to be more prevalent during middle age and older. These statistics may be linked with age-related obstructive sleep disorders such as snoring and hypopnea and may be the cause of subclinical hypoxia.

Hypnic headaches are characterised by varying degrees of head pain, ranging from mild to severe. Fortunately, these headaches can often be easily alleviated through simple measures such as rising and enjoying a cup of coffee or practicing mindful breathing. However, discerning between a hypnic headache and a migraine headache poses a challenge based on clinical observations and personal experiences. Some morning headaches, initially perceived as benign, have the potential to evolve into full-fledged migraines over the course of the day. This is especially challenging for individuals like me who are hesitant to resort to medication and prefer to wait and observe. However, over the years, I have noticed one discerning method to differentiate between a hypnic headache and a migraine is to pay attention to your dreams. If you experience vivid, adventurous or nightmarish dreams, these, along with other premonition symptoms unique to you, serve as a forewarning of an impending migraine.

While the research landscape continues to grapple with the complex nature of the causes behind early morning headaches, the naturopathic approach considers the homeostasis of cerebral tissue and its continuum to maintain optimal function. Disruption to this delicate balance can arise from an array of influences encompassing inflammation, oxidative stress, nutrient deficiencies, disturbances in electrolytes, and glucose metabolism. Among these factors, insufficient tissue oxygenation emerges as a pivotal element deserving a more in-depth discussion. In the following section, we will delve extensively into the intricate dynamics of tissue oxygenation and its profound implications on cerebral function.

Overall, these disturbances collectively lay the groundwork for a heightened vulnerability and reactivity in cerebral tissue and therefore increased susceptibility to headaches and migraines.

I need to add that there are other potential causes of early morning headaches, such as dehydration, medication side effects, alcohol consumption, etc. It is important to consult with a naturopathic clinician for a thorough evaluation and perform the necessary assessments to determine the specific underlying issues.

While shallow breathing is not recognised as a direct cause of migraines, it is acknowledged that it can alter blood oxygen levels.[147] Therefore, shallow breathing and the resulting subclinical hypoxia can be an underlying trigger for early morning headaches and migraines. This scenario is physiologically plausible, as the neuropeptide hypocretin (orexin) plays a significant role in awakening from sleep, particularly in response to decreased oxygen levels. Orexin triggers the rapid release of glutamate,[148] a molecule known to alter vascular tone, activate inflammatory molecules, and transmit pain.

Breathing is intricately connected to the functioning of the nervous system, and you have the unique ability to regulate your stress response and improve oxygenation by cultivating mindful breathing habits.

Bringing awareness to your breathing patterns will help you to promote and practice deep abdominal breathing. Diaphragmatic or belly breathing can help maximise lung capacity, improve oxygenation, and promote a relaxation response through activation of the vagus nerve.

The vagus nerve is a key component of the parasympathetic nervous system, which is responsible for the body's 'rest and digest' functions. The smooth muscles of the bronchi and bronchioles in the lungs are directly influenced by vagal activity, leading to relaxation of these muscles. This process, known as bronchodilation, results in increased airflow into the lungs, enhanced cardiovascular flow, and improved oxygen uptake. When activity of the vagus nerve is restored, it can help reduce stress and anxiety levels, lower blood pressure, and promote a sense of calm.

The restoration of vagal activity also strengthens respiratory muscles for efficient breathing. While insufficient physical activity might not directly lead to shallow breathing, it can contribute to respiratory and cardiovascular problems, ultimately affecting breathing efficiency. Engaging in regular physical activity improves lung capacity, strengthens respiratory muscles and enhances overall cardiovascular fitness, facilitating efficient oxygen delivery to body tissues. Cultivating healthier breathing patterns can reduce stress, promote more restful sleep, and lead to fewer headaches and migraines.

Brain Bites and Guided Strategies

- Hypoxia is the condition in which the body is deprived of adequate oxygen delivery to its tissues. Several studies have validated that hypoxia can trigger or exacerbate migraines, especially in cortical spreading depression (CSD) and visual aura.

- Obstructive sleep disorders such as snoring, hypopnea and apnoea can lead to subclinical hypoxia.

- Subclinical hypoxia is intricately connected with stress, shallow breathing and sleep disordered breathing.

Understanding the role of hypoxia in migraines can offer insights into potential management strategies, particularly for those with shallow breathing and sleep disordered breathing. The following protocols provide specific strategies to help with shallow breathing and increase the efficiency of oxygen delivery to body and brain tissue.

The following strategies can be found in The Therapy Kit, Chapter 5, Section 5.8.

1. The Vagal Breathing Method is a breathing technique that stimulates the vagus nerve and can improve breathing habits and reduce stress. Refer to Subsection 5.8.1.

2. Nutrient strategies to manage stress. Refer to Subsection 5.8.3.

3. Improving lung capacity and strengthening diaphragm muscles enhances respiratory function. Refer to Subsection 5.8.2.

4. Addressing sleep apnoea and other breathing disorders. Refer to Section 5.5.

4.10 The Power of Sunlight

You have already learned about various strategies for supporting healthy serotonin levels, understanding how this essential neurotransmitter impacts mood, wellbeing and the susceptibility to migraines. One other way to boost serotonin is through sunlight exposure. Numerous studies show that exposure to natural sunlight, particularly in the morning, is crucial for maintaining healthy serotonin levels. When sunlight reaches the retina in the eyes, it boosts the brain chemical serotonin and helps us feel more alert. It also keeps our sleep cycle regular and assists in maintaining mood and energy.

One thing we may need to consider is the use of sunglasses. While sunglasses are undoubtedly valuable for eye protection, frequent use, especially dark sunglasses, may block the beneficial blue light that stimulates serotonin production.

While there is no specific research on the effects of sunglasses on serotonin levels, there is substantial research on the effects of sunlight exposure, or lack thereof. Even cloudy days have been shown to affect serotonin when compared to sunny days, highlighting the potential benefits of natural light for wellbeing.[149,150]

Additionally, serotonin is also a precursor for melatonin, the hormone that helps regulate sleep. Reduced light exposure due to sunglasses could disrupt the body's internal clock, leading to difficulties with sleep. This can in turn make it harder to maintain a regular sleep schedule, which can further affect serotonin levels.[151]

Nordic populations, living in areas with limited sunlight during the winter months, commonly experience Seasonal Affective Disorder (SAD) and Vitamin D deficiency. The lack of sunlight disrupts their natural serotonin and melatonin balance, leading to symptoms of SAD, such as low energy, mood swings and sleep disturbances. Additionally, insufficient sunlight prevents the body from producing adequate Vitamin D.[152]

Vitamin D is an important link between natural sunlight and optimal serotonin production. Known as the 'sunshine vitamin', it is produced in the skin in response to sunlight. This vitamin plays a distinct yet complementary role in supporting serotonin production. Vitamin D regulates the expression of tryptophan hydroxylase 2 (TPH2), an enzyme that converts the amino acid tryptophan into serotonin. Adequate vitamin D levels help ensure that serotonin production occurs efficiently. In contrast, low vitamin D levels may reduce TPH2 expression, potentially leading to decreased serotonin production.[153]

In summary, while sunglasses are essential for eye protection, frequent use may slightly impact serotonin and melatonin balance, which can be a trigger for those prone to migraines. Moderating sunglasses use, especially during morning light exposure, might help support mood, sleep and wellbeing in sensitive individuals.

Brain Bites and Guided Strategies

- Optimal serotonin levels require daily exposure to sunlight.

- Vitamin D is synthesised from sunlight and plays a crucial role in serotonin production.

- To maximise benefits from morning sunlight, refrain from wearing sunglasses.

The following strategies and treatment options can be found in The Therapy Kit, Chapter 5.

- Treat yourself to regular morning sunlight to promote the production of vitamin D and serotonin. For more information on vitamin D, refer to Subsection 5.7.4.

CHAPTER 5

The Therapy Kit

Treatment Strategies

The treatments and strategies presented in this book have been carefully chosen for their proven effectiveness in reducing the frequency and severity of migraines. However, to unlock their full potential, it is crucial to follow these approaches with commitment and dedication. These therapies are not just tools to be tried, they are part of a thoughtfully designed pathway to facilitate genuine healing and restore systemic vitality. The strategies aim to reduce tissue sensitivities and target the root causes that contribute to the inflammatory pathways leading to migraines.

To help you benefit from these treatments, I highly recommend reaching out for professional support, especially in the areas of herbal medicine and nutritional supplementation. These medical interventions are often best navigated with the insight of an experienced practitioner. A naturopath or qualified health professional can guide you through this process and help tailor a personalised plan to meet your specific needs.

The healing process from migraines is a journey of reducing systemic sensitivities, cultivating resilience and regaining vitality. Investing in professional support is not just about getting advice; it's about empowering yourself with the knowledge and expertise necessary to achieve lasting results. Your journey towards better health deserves the best guidance available.

Please keep in mind that this book is intended for informational purposes only. It is not a substitute for professional medical advice, diagnosis, or treatment. Always seek the advice of your physician or other qualified healthcare provider with any questions you may have regarding a medical condition. The authors and publisher are not responsible for any errors or omissions or for any outcomes related to the use of this material.

5.1 Making Use of the Migraine Trigger Checklist for Effective Diary use

Before you embark on your diary-tracking journey, it is essential to familiarise yourself with the list of migraine triggers, including dietary, lifestyle and environmental factors. Take a reflective moment to see if any of these may be potential triggers for you. This process will help you identify recurring patterns in your daily habits and environment more easily.

I have compiled a list of common migraine triggers below to get you started on your journey to better migraine management. Keep in mind that migraine triggers vary greatly from person to person, so it is essential to personalise your diary based on your unique experiences. By diligently tracking your triggers and learning to avoid these, you will begin to observe a shift in the frequency and severity of your migraines.

5.2 List of External and Internal Triggers

In Chapter 2, you learned how to identify triggers and their characteristics. You also learned that migraines can be triggered by a wide range of factors, both external and internal, and can vary greatly from one individual to another.

External triggers often involve environmental or lifestyle factors, such as diet, physical activity and exposure to certain stimuli, while internal triggers pertain to physiological processes within the body, including hormonal fluctuations, dehydration and sleep disturbances.

This section outlines a comprehensive list of external and internal triggers, along with references to chapters that provide further detail on how these factors may influence migraine onset. The triggers presented here serve as a guide to help recognise potential contributors.

External Triggers

Food compounds

- Amines, glutamate, nitrites, citric acid, and alcoholic beverages (Chapter 3). While there are only a few compounds that act as a trigger for migraines, they are widely distributed across various foods. Therefore, I have provided a separate food list indicating where these compounds are present. The list can be found in Chapter 5, Section 5.3.

Food intolerance or allergies

- Excess histamine can lead to an inflammatory process and activates the trigeminovascular system. If you would like more information on this topic, go to Chapter 3, Section 3.4.

Poor posture

- Poor workstation ergonomics or standing or sitting in the same position for prolonged periods leads to muscle fatigue and spasms. You can find more information on this topic in Chapter 4, Sections 2.1 and 2.4.

Teeth grinding or clenching

- This typically occurs during the night and can serve as an early warning sign (premonition phase). This stress-induced activity directly impacts the trigeminal nerve and activates the trigeminovascular system.

Strenuous physical activity and physical exertion

- Engaging in excessive or strenuous exercises or physical labour, particularly in hot climates, can lead to several migraine triggers, including overheating, dehydration and electrolyte imbalances. You can find more information on this topic in Chapter 2, Section 2.4 and Chapter 4, Section 4.3.

Lighting

- Exposure to bright, dim or flickering light from artificial or fluorescent lights and computer screens. This affects the mood leading to irritation or short temper and symptoms such as sore eyes, fatigue, a foggy mind, or tension headaches.

Odours

- Distinctive smells which are mostly regarded as unpleasant. This can include perfumes, cigarette smoke, strong chemicals, household cleaners, synthetic air fresheners, diesel fumes, and fumes from incinerators and bushfires, etc. Odours are personal and may even be quite bothersome to some individuals and instantly recognised as potential triggers.

Weather

- Windy weather and atmospheric pressure influence positive ions. For some individuals, windy weather can be bothersome and affect mood and can also be a potential premonition phase.

Perceived stress

- Mental stress leads to a biological process in the body called the fight or flight response, and a shift in neurotransmitters. You can find more information on this topic in Chapter 4, Section 4.2.

Fasting or skipping meals

- Fasting or skipping meals can be risky for people with blood sugar regulation problems as it may lead to hypoglycemia or electrolyte imbalances and trigger a stress response. For more information on blood sugar regulation, go to Chapter 3 'Hypoglycemia' (Section 3.9).

Internal Triggers

Adrenalin rush

- This signifies a significant neurotransmitter shift associated with the fight-or-flight response. One notable thing is that you become acutely aware of your heart pounding towards the end of the adrenalin rush. Some examples that can influence an adrenalin rush include bungy jumping, sudden falls or stumbles, the heightened arousal during an orgasm, witnessing an accident, or engaging in confrontations marked by heightened aggression.

Dehydration

- Dehydration occurs when the body loses more fluids than it takes in, leading to an insufficient amount of water to carry out normal bodily functions. It can result from excessive sweating, vomiting, diarrhoea, or insufficient fluid intake. Symptoms include thirst, dry mouth, dizziness, and fatigue. However, what tends to be more common is subclinical dehydration. This is mild and often unnoticed, where fluid loss is not severe enough to cause obvious symptoms but can still affect the body's normal functioning. It may lead to fatigue, reduced cognitive performance or decreased physical endurance and over time, it can increase the risk of more serious dehydration or health issues. It often occurs due to inadequate daily water intake. Optimal fluid levels are essential for the movement of electrolytes, which is critical for proper cellular function.

Electrolyte imbalances

- Electrolytes are essential minerals (ions) in the body that help conduct electrical impulses necessary for various physiological processes, including fluid balance, nerve function and muscle contraction and relaxation. These processes are particularly relevant to migraine susceptibility. Electrolyte imbalances, especially involving sodium chloride (salt) and magnesium, can result from factors such as dehydration, fasting, diarrhoea, and nutrient deficiencies.

Hormonal changes

- Hormonal fluctuations or changes such as those that occur during menstruation, menopause and hormone therapy. For more information, go to Chapter 3, Section 3.8.

Sleep disturbances

- Lack of sleep and changes in sleep patterns can affect neurotransmitter balance.

Subclinical hypoxia

- Subtle oxygen deprivation in brain tissue. You can find information on this topic in Chapter 4, Sections 4.7 and 4.8.

5.3 List of Top Foods that can Trigger Migraines

The following list includes a specific selection of foods that are commonly associated with migraine triggers, based on clinical evidence and patient-reported experiences. To make it easy to navigate, the table is organised by food groups and sorted alphabetically within each group. Each food entry is also marked with a key for specific triggers (e.g. 'G' for glutamate, 'H' for histamine, etc), allowing quick reference to relevant compounds. Additionally, a notes section provides extra information on specific foods where applicable.

A few pointers to keep in mind:

- Amine levels can vary significantly in fresh produce, largely depending on how fresh they are. These variations can make it challenging to detect patterns and potential triggers when reviewing your food diary.

- High putrescine (P) foods may potentially interfere with histamine levels, causing symptoms similar to histamine intolerance.

- Cumulative response occurs when more than one trigger compound is present in a single food, or when a meal includes multiple foods containing trigger compounds, leading to an intensified or additive trigger response.

Key

G - Glutamate or MSG
H - Histamine
N - Nitrates
P - Putrescine
T - Tyramine
V - Vanilloid receptor
C – Citric Acid

Food Type	Trigger Compounds	Additional Comments on Specific Foods
The food additive Glutamate. *Check ingredient labels carefully.	G	Glutamate comes in many forms, including *Monopotassium Glutamate* (E 622), *Calcium Glutamate* (E 623), *Monoammonium Glutamate* (E 624), and the most used *Monosodium Glutamate* (MSG), (E 621). As MSG is viewed unfavourably by some consumers, food companies often avoid using the term 'MSG' on ingredient

Found in most ready packet sauces & meals Deli meats Savoury biscuits	G G G G	labels and instead use terms like 'natural flavours', 'flavouring' or 'flavour enhancer'. For more information on glutamate in food, refer to Chapter 3, Section 3.7. Glutamate is present in a wide variety of savoury and sweet foods, including chips, snacks, pizzas, ready-to-eat meals, meat products, instant soups, charcuterie meats, tinned foods, and milk chocolate. Magnesium Glutamate (E 625) is rarely used except in low sodium meat products. Yeast Extract (E620) is added to some foods like soy sauce and cheese for a savory flavour. Also found in canned soups and stews, frozen dinners and salty snacks. Gelatine (E441) obtained from animal products. The gelatine is highly processed and can contain around 8-9 grams per 100g.
BEVERAGES		
Alcohol (ethanol)	V	Vanilloid 1 receptor (TRPV1) functions as a sensory monitor in the walls of blood vessels and reacts to any anomalies in the blood it deems as noxious. It also triggers vasodilation and inflammation.
Orange juice	P, C	Fruit juice contains particularly high levels of putrescine,
Mandarin juice	P, C	
Grapefruit juice	P, C	
Red wine	H, T, V,	
Soybean milk	P	Negligible amounts, depending on amount consumed.
Soft drinks	G, C	Many soft drinks, including tonic water, contain glutamate with the terms 'natural flavours', 'flavouring'.
Cordials	G, C	

CONDIMENTS		
Fish sauce Tomato paste Ketchup Soy sauce Worcestershire sauce	G G G, C G G	These products are naturally high in glutamate and may also have glutamate additive to enhance flavour.
DAIRY PRODUCTS		
Hard Cheese: Parmesan Cheddar Gouda	G, H, T G, H, T G, H, T G, H, T	Hard cheeses are dense, which means they contain more protein. More protein results in greater production of glutamate, tyramine and histamine during aging, increasing the potential for triggering symptoms.
Soft Cheese: Brie Camembert Gorgonzola Roquefort Blue cheese	G, H, T G, H, T G, H, T G, H, T G, H, T	Soft cheeses generally contain less protein, resulting in lower amounts of these compounds. However, certain aged soft cheeses can still produce enough glutamate, tyramine and histamine to be a concern.
FRUIT		
Bananas	P	
Oranges	P, C	Fresh and unprocessed oranges have incremental amounts of putrescine.
Grapefruit	T, P, C	
Lemons & Limes	C	
Purple Passionfruit	P, C	
Watermelon	N	More likely a trigger if eaten in large amounts.

MEATS		
Pork roast, chops, sausages	G H H, G, N	Unlike other animal proteins, pork has natural but unusually high amino acids of histidine and glutamic acid both in the lean meat and fat. This will produce histamine and glutamate during cooking and storage.
Chicken	H, T	Increases with processing, storage, cooking, leftovers.
Bacon	H, G, N	
Ham	H, G, N	
Pastrami	H, G, N	
Fish	H, G, T, P	Increases with storage, freezing, cooking, and kept as leftovers.
shellfish	H, G, T, P	Increases with storage, freezing, cooking, and kept as leftovers.
GRAINS		
Rice	G	Grains like rice and wheat contain approximately 10 to 16 mg of bound glutamate, and the cooking process for these grains generally poses no concern. However, I have had a small number of patients who seem to react to white rice, but only if it is extensively cooked in fluids, such as risotto.
NUTS		
Walnuts	G	658 mg of glutamate per 100 grams. Be aware of walnut butter.
Pistachio	P	
Peanuts	G	5243 mg of glutamate per 100 grams. Be aware of peanut butter.

SWEETS		
Ice-creams	G	Some ice creams have MSG. This may be labelled as 'food additive 621' or 'flavour enhancer 621' natural flavour.
Chocolate	G	Ingredient labels will use terms like 'natural flavours', 'flavouring'.
VEGETABLES		Concentration of amines vary greatly and depend on freshness and storage time of vegetable products.
Asparagus	H, T	
Aubergine	H, T	
Avocado	G, H, T	The active compounds are relatively low compared to foods like tomatoes or cheese, and since avocado is typically eaten raw, most migraine sufferers do not react adversely to it.
Chard	T	
Corn	G, P	
Capsicum	G	
Kelp dried	G	
Mushrooms	G, P	
Peas	G, P	
Peppers Green	P	
Soybeans	P	
Soybean sprouts	P	
Spinach	H, T, N	
Tomatoes	H, G, T	The tomato pulp contains the highest amount of glutamate with an average of 140-250 mg per 100 grams of tomato. The cherry tomato is the most potent of all tomatoes.
Wheat germ	P	

| Ginger | V | Some highly sensitive individuals react to both ginger and capsaicin, as both activate the vanilloid receptors. These receptors function as a sensory monitor in the walls of blood vessels and react to any anomalies in the blood they deem as noxious. They also trigger vasodilation and inflammation. |
| Chili peppers | V | Capsaicin. |

5.4 The Migraine Diary

Managing and preventing migraines begins with understanding that your migraine journey is uniquely yours. Only you possess the personal knowledge and bodily insight needed to overcome your migraines, making you your greatest asset. The migraine diary is your most powerful tool in this journey, enabling you to uncover patterns, pinpoint triggers and make meaningful connections that only you can identify. The migraine diary is more than just a tool for management; it is the ultimate self-empowering tool that can help you conquer migraines once and for all.

To get started, simply visit my website at www.lilliclemens.com and under the tools tab you can access the migraine diary template. With its easy-to-use electronic format, the form will walk you through each section with select options, making it quick and simple to log important information like daily stressors, sleep quality, food intake, and other factors that may play a part in your migraines. Daily use will help you identify trends and triggers, empowering you to take control of your migraine management and work towards lasting relief.

5.5 Sleep Disordered Breathing

The primary goal of treating sleep-disordered breathing is to improve and maintain adequate oxygen levels in the brain. This helps to prevent inflammation and reduce the likelihood of experiencing morning migraines. The following treatments will be specifically based on obstructive disordered breathing (SDB) and shallow breathing (hypopnea). If you would like to know more about these conditions, go to Chapter 4 in Sections 4.7, 4.8 and 4.9.

5.5.1 Obstructive Disordered Breathing (SDB)

- There are several treatments available for obstructive SDB depending on the severity of the disorder. Firstly, you need to make an appointment with your physician to organise a sleep study. You can now do this study in the comfort of your own home with a small sleep testing device that will monitor and record oxygen saturation, blood pressure and frequency in waking and snoring.

- In your return visit, your sleep data will be analysed, and the health provider will discuss and provide you with several options in how to improve your oxygen saturation and sleep.

- For severe apnoea, you may be advised to use a CPAP machine, which provides a continuous positive air pressure to keep the airway open. Another option to keep the airways open and reduce snoring is the use of a mandibular splint, which is a type of night mouth guard that helps to reposition the lower jaw during sleep.

- If your diagnosis is a mild obstructive SDB, then a mandibular splint is all you may need. Alternatively, there are also lifestyle choices you can implement to reduce the severity and frequency of SDB. The natural alternatives to improve sleep and oxygen saturation are fundamentally the most advantageous course of treatment for long term and you will find the following treatment options helpful in making an informed choice.

Some natural treatments you can put into practice are as follows:

5.5.2 Side Sleeping

- Snoring is not a condition that is easily resolved and as we grow older, snoring may increase. However, what we can do is consciously implement some strategies that will help to reduce the frequency and duration of snoring and provide a good night's sleep overall.

- Since the tongue is often the main cause of reduced air movement, a good strategy to keep the airway open is to practice sleeping on your side instead of your back. To enhance comfort while sleeping on your side, it is recommended to use a pillow to support your back or place a firm pillow between your knees. A knee pillow is particularly important if you suffer from lower back pain as it improves comfort and reduces pain. When choosing a mattress for side sleeping, opt for a medium to firm mattress that contours to your body's shape. Keep in mind that side sleeping may take some time to get used to, but comfort is key to making it a successful practice.

5.5.3 Alcohol Consumption

- Unfortunately, consuming alcoholic drinks in the evening is not advisable if you are already susceptible to Sleep-Disordered Breathing (SDB). After a few drinks, your airway and tongue may relax just as much as you do. Later, when you are in a deep sleep, this relaxation can lead to your airway vibrating throughout the night, resulting in disrupted sleep, and potentially worsening your condition.

- Yes, it is a tough decision. After a busy, stressful day, there's nothing more tempting than unwinding with a glass of something special alongside your dinner. However, this decision ultimately revolves around your long-term health. As the Billy Ocean song goes, 'When the going gets tough, the tough get going.'

- For many, trying to reduce alcohol consumption too quickly often leads to failure. Each subsequent attempt can become more challenging as abrupt changes can significantly affect your mood, increasing the temptation to reach for a drink. That's why it is important to reduce alcohol gradually and incrementally, allowing your body to acclimate.

- The first step is to create a plan (see example below) that outlines how you will slowly decrease your evening alcohol intake, along with a target date for achieving this goal. This plan should be visual, easily accessible and placed in a prominent spot, such as on the fridge, where you can check off your progress day by day.

- To validate the positive changes using the Alcohol Planner, you will need to track your daily moods, sleep and any headache or migraine symptoms in the Migraine Diary.

WEEKLY PLANNER TO REDUCE ALCOHOL CONSUMPTION

The strategy is to adhere to a weekly reduction plan with a stop date.

Over a period of four weeks, gradually reduce the number of drinks. The portion of alcoholic drink removed is replaced with an alternative.

Date Started:

Week 1 remove ¼ of usual alcohol intake
Day 1 ☐ Day 2 ☐ Day 3 ☐ Day 4 ☐ Day 5 ☐ Day 6 ☐ Day 7 ☐

Week 2 remove ½ of usual alcohol intake
Day 1 ☐ Day 2 ☐ Day 3 ☐ Day 4 ☐ Day 5 ☐ Day 6 ☐ Day 7 ☐

Week 3 remove ¾ of usual alcohol intake
Day 1 ☐ Day 2 ☐ Day 3 ☐ Day 4 ☐ Day 5 ☐ Day 6 ☐ Day 7 ☐

Week 4 alcohol free
Day 1 ☐ Day 2 ☐ Day 3 ☐ Day 4 ☐ Day 5 ☐ Day 6 ☐ Day 7 ☐

Alternative replacements: add sparkling water or soda to your beverage, space the time between each drink, and take smaller sips to make it last.

Avoid thirst when you drink and have a glass of sparkling water between drinks.

Alternatives to alcohol

- Alcohol-free beverages are all the rage these days, and you will likely find your local supermarket stocked with a wide variety, including sparkling wines, beers and even spirits like gin and vodka—all without the alcohol. Just make sure to check the ingredient labels as these may contain glutamate, citric acid and other potential trigger compounds. If you are interested in crafting some stylish and sophisticated alcohol-free drinks and cocktails at home, you might want to explore Julia Bainbridge's book, *Good Drinks: Alcohol-Free Recipes for When You're Not Drinking for Whatever Reason.* It offers a range of creative recipes perfect for any occasion.

For those looking to rethink their relationship with alcohol, *Mindful Drinking: How Cutting Down Can Change Your Life* by Rosamund Dean is another excellent resource. This book provides insightful guidance on how to reduce your alcohol intake while still enjoying a vibrant social life.

5.5.4 Weight Loss

- Carrying excess body weight can significantly affect your sleep quality and overall health. Extra fatty tissue around the throat and neck can exacerbate shortness of breath (SOB), particularly during sleep. Numerous studies highlight the benefits of weight loss in reducing SOB and enhancing sleep quality. For personalised advice and a tailored weight loss plan, consult your healthcare provider.

5.5.5 Diaphragmatic Breathing Exercise

- When you are stressed or mentally preoccupied, you tend to breathe shallowly, limiting lung capacity and reducing oxygen intake. To counteract this, I recommend practising diaphragmatic breathing twice a day for five minutes per session. You can perform this exercise while sitting in a chair or lying down in a quiet, comfortable place.

Personally, I find it beneficial to do my breathing exercises in bed before sleeping and again in the morning upon waking. Additionally, you can use apps like *Fitbit* or *Apple Watch* for guided breathing exercises, or download apps such as *Breathe2Relax* or *Oak - Meditation & Breathing* to support your routine.

This exercise is designed to enhance oxygen intake, strengthen your diaphragm and reduce stress.

Step 1: Find a Comfortable Position

- **Option 1** - Sit in a chair with your feet flat on the floor, back straight.

- **Option 2** - Lie down on your back with your knees bent and your head supported by a pillow. Place a pillow under your knees for extra support if needed.

Step 2: Place Your Hands

- Place one hand on your chest and the other on your abdomen, just below your ribcage. This will help you feel the movement of your diaphragm as you breathe.

Step 3: Breathe In

- Inhale slowly and deeply through your nose, allowing your abdomen to rise as your lungs fill with air. You should feel the hand on your abdomen rise, while the hand on your chest should remain relatively still.

Step 4: Breathe Out

- Exhale steadily through pursed lips (as if you're blowing out a candle), feeling your hand on your abdomen fall, while the hand on your chest stays still. The exhale should last longer than the inhale as you gently push out that little extra air from your lungs without straining.

Step 5: Establish a Rhythm

- Continue this breathing pattern for about five minutes, focusing on making each breath steady, deep and controlled. Relax your shoulders and maintain a steady rhythm.

Step 6: Practice Regularly

- Aim to practice diaphragmatic breathing twice a day—once in the morning when you wake up and again before you go to sleep. Each session should last a minimum of five minutes.

5.6 Trigeminal Dysphoria and Eye Strain

Maintaining good eye health is crucial, especially in the digital age where prolonged screen time can lead to issues such as trigeminal dysphoria and eye strain. Below are some effective methods to help alleviate these symptoms and strengthen your vision.

Exercises for Eye Health

Ideally, we should take a break from the computer screen at least every 40 minutes. Simply getting up for a walk and using your long-distance vision gives the delicate muscles of the eyes a chance to rest and recover. Additionally, blinking intentionally during breaks can help keep your eyes moist and prevent dryness, which is common with prolonged screen use. Ensuring your workspace is well-lit and adjusting screen brightness to match your environment can further reduce strain on your eyes.

1. Near & Far Focus Exercise

- Focusing is a vital aspect of vision, and regular exercises can enhance this ability, allowing you to rely more confidently on your eyesight. Here's how to perform a simple focusing exercise:

  Step 1: Choose an object approximately 10 to 20 metres away.

Step 2: Extend your arm and hold your thumb upright in front of you.

Step 3: Shift your focus from your thumb to the distant object and back again.

Step 4: Repeat this process five times.

This exercise helps train your eyes to adjust between near and far distances, which can reduce eye strain and improve overall focus.

2. Palming

- The palming technique is a simple and effective method to relax your eyes and reduce eye strain. This technique is particularly useful for those who spend long hours in front of screens or experience stress-related eye discomfort. Here's how to perform the palming exercise.

Follow these simple Steps

- **Find a comfortable position:** Sit in a comfortable chair or at a desk with your elbows resting on a flat surface. You can also sit cross-legged on the floor with your elbows resting on your knees.

- **Warm your hands:** Rub your palms together briskly until they feel warm. The warmth generated by this friction will help soothe your eyes.

- **Cover your eyes:** Gently cup your hands over your closed eyes. Make sure not to press on your eyelids; your hands should just rest lightly on your face. Your fingers should be placed on your forehead, and the base of your palms should cover the cheekbones. This creates a dark, relaxing environment for your eyes.

- **Relax and breathe:** Close your eyes and take deep, slow breaths. Focus on your breathing and allow yourself to relax completely. Visualise darkness or a calming scene while your eyes are covered. This helps to relax your eye muscles mentally and physically.

- **Hold the position:** Stay in this position for one to three minutes, or longer if you feel particularly stressed. The longer you hold the position, the more relaxed your eyes will feel.

- **Slowly uncover your eyes:** After the time has passed, slowly lower your hands, and open your eyes. Take a moment to adjust to the light before resuming your activities.

5.7 The Top 4 Must-Have Nutrients to Combat Migraine

I believe it is essential to dedicate a special section to certain key nutrients that are central in this discussion. These nutrients are not only crucial for many of the biochemical pathways affected by migraines but also commonly found to be deficient in migraine sufferers. Their deficiency can significantly impact the therapeutic outcome in relieving migraines. You will find that these nutrients are also discussed in other parts of this book, highlighting their multiple important roles in the body.

The nutrients you will find in this section are essential and often deficient in individuals with migraines. Below, each nutrient is listed with reasons for its importance, recommended therapeutic dosage, and available dietary sources.

I have only provided the therapeutic dosage ranges for these nutrients as the actual dosages should be determined by your clinical practitioner. The genetic and physiological diversity in nutrient needs is highly individual and the nutritional requirements depend on the individual's rate of absorption, metabolism, excretion, and dietary strategies. Therefore, the following therapeutic dosages recommendations are a guide only.

It is important to note that supplemental nutrients should generally be considered for short term, to help address deficiencies and facilitate rapid recovery, especially when dealing with food intolerance and food avoidance during the healing journey.

Essentially, these nutrients are naturally present in foods, offering a more optimal synergistic utilisation and therapeutic effect compared to supplements. Therefore, dietary advice becomes not only more sustainable but also more clinically beneficial.

I strongly recommend that you see a naturopathic practitioner to help you identify any specific nutrient deficiencies you may have and determine the specific therapeutic dosages you will need. All nutrient therapies described in this book require supervision by an experienced healthcare professional.

5.7.1 5-HTP (5-hydroxytryptophan)

Prescription: 50-70mg, once daily.

Administration: Sublingual (powder form)

Instructions:

- Preferable to take first thing in the morning before food.

- Avoid swallowing the powder to ensure optimal absorption via oral mucosa.

- Store the medication in a cool, dry place, away from direct sunlight.

- Follow up with your healthcare provider regularly to monitor your response to the medication.

Mode of action:

- The primary mechanism of 5-HTP is to increase levels of serotonin in the central nervous system (brain and spinal cord).

- Positive effects of 5-HTP on other neurotransmitters include melatonin. This neurotransmitter improves sleep quality and helps with sleep disorders. It also increases levels of beta-endorphin, opioid compounds that aid in pain relief; regulates inflammatory response; reduces stress; and improves mental health.[154]

Caution:

- There is some anecdotal evidence that 5-HTP should not be used for acute migraine treatment, as it has been observed that some individuals have experienced mild serotonin syndrome symptoms, including flushing, nausea, and tachycardia.

- 5-HTP is recommended only for patients with chronic stress, anxiety, or depression.

- It is suggested that 5-HTP should be used with caution in patients taking SSRI or MAOI antidepressants. Although several observational studies have examined the combination of MAOI antidepressants and 5-HTP at a dosage of around 300 mg per day, no evidence of serotonin syndrome was observed.[155,156] However, caution is still warranted as sublingual administration has a higher availability.

Notes:

5-Hydroxytryptophan, commonly known as 5-HTP is a supplement I recommend for patients experiencing chronic stress, anxiety, or depression. 5-HTP is a natural compound that your body synthesises from the amino acid L-tryptophan to produce serotonin. The commercial form of 5-HTP is a naturally derived product from the seeds of the African plant Griffonia simplicifolia.[157] Therapeutically, it has an amazing ability to boost serotonin levels in the brain.

The added benefit of 5-HTP is that it serves as a direct pathway to serotonin production. Unlike L-tryptophan, 5-HTP is not diverted into producing other compounds like niacin or proteins; it directly contributes to serotonin synthesis.

Your body absorbs 5-HTP easily without needing special transport molecules. Additionally, 5-HTP easily crosses the blood-brain barrier, making it an effective way to increase brain serotonin levels.

Although prescriptions for 5-HTP are generally via the oral route, I have found that sublingual (under the tongue) administration is more effective. Here is why:

Oral administration means that 5-HTP must be absorbed via digestion, but this has its challenges. Firstly, the typical dosage is generally between 200-500 mg per day to make it therapeutically effective. Much of the 5-HTP is converted to serotonin in the digestive system and other peripheral parts of the body.[27] It is important to note that the high dosages often lead to side effects with symptoms of nausea, vomiting and diarrhoea.

In comparison, sublingual administration of 5-HTP is more effective, offering faster absorption directly into the blood stream, with a higher bioavailability, allowing for smaller doses, with fewer side effects.

5.7.2 Magnesium

Prescription: Therapeutic dosage for migraine prevention 300-500 mg/day.

Administration: oral administration away from food.

Instructions:

- The therapeutic dosage should be taken for approximately 2 months, after which it should be reduced to a daily maintenance dosage of approximately 100-300 mg. Both the therapeutic dosage and maintenance dosage is highly dependent on individual needs, the state of migraine pathology, gender, age, and dietary intake.

- I would recommend an organic magnesium compound as these have better bioavailability. This would include Magnesium citrate, Magnesium glycinate or Magnesium L-threonate, all of which have high bioavailability, meaning more of the magnesium is absorbed and available to have an active effect in the body.

- If the therapeutic recommended dose is above 200 mg, consider dividing the dosage into two or three times per day to improve efficiency of the nutrient.

- High doses of magnesium should not be taken with food due to its alkaline nature, which can adversely affect stomach acidity and consequently food absorption.

Notes:

Magnesium is a multifunctional mineral essential for brain function and regulation. The following points illustrate its importance in migraine pathology:

- Migraine sufferers are commonly magnesium deficient.

- Although magnesium does not have a direct analgesic effect (pain relief), it blocks the sensation of pain (antinociceptive effect) by occupying NMDA receptors, which inhibits calcium ions from entering cells.[158] Magnesium is a NMDA receptor antagonist which helps to regulate glutamate activity, [159] reduce pain transmission and inhibit the activity of vasoactive chemicals such as substance P and CGRP.[160] From this perspective, magnesium has the unique ability to dampen the neuronal hyperexcitability characteristic of migraine sufferers.[161]

- Magnesium is also a GABA receptor agonist. It activates the GBA receptor to produce a calming effect, by reducing stress and anxiety.[161]

- Magnesium combats oxidative stress (acting as an antioxidant) and inflammation, and relaxes blood vessels via smooth muscle activity[160]

- Magnesium plays a role in protecting the structural integrity and function of the blood-brain barrier.[160] This protection prevents the entry of toxins and other infectious material, which can lead to inflammation and oxidative stress.

- As a cofactor, magnesium is needed for the conversion of tryptophan to 5-hydroxytryptophan (5-HTP) in the serotonin pathway[162] and for the production of GABA[161] the calming neurotransmitter.

- Magnesium enhances neuronal plasticity.[160] This aids the healing capacity of a migraine brain and improves the brain's resilience to migraine triggers.

Caution:

- Magnesium is poorly absorbed due to the following factors. Vitamin D deficiency, the use of proton pump inhibitors, diarrhoea, bowel disease, and laxative use.

- Increased kidney loss of magnesium may occur with diabetes, drug use and alcohol.[162]

- Supplementary citrate can trigger migraines and headaches in some individuals. To avoid this, opt for alternatives like magnesium glycinate or zinc glycinate instead of magnesium citrate or zinc citrate supplements.

Dietary sources:

Magnesium is available across all natural foods, but some are particularly magnesium rich in the following examples.

- Vegetables – spinach, Swiss chard, kale, cabbage, all green leafy vegetables, kelp, potatoes with skin, broccoli, green beans, sweet corn, green peas, parsnips.

- Fruit – avocado, papaya, figs, dates, kiwi, raisins, passion fruit, raspberries, blackberry, bananas, cantaloupe, watermelon, mango, apricots, cherries, pineapple, oranges, rhubarb, and mandarins.

- Nuts and seeds – almonds, hazelnuts, Brazil nuts, cashews, hemp, brown rice, quinoa, and buckwheat.

5.7.3 Zinc

Prescription: 0.2 mg per kg of body weight once daily.

Administration: oral

Instructions:

- Take with food to avoid stomach upset (preferably a protein source).

- I recommend zinc picolinate, zinc citrate and zinc glycinate for best absorption and bioavailability.

Notes:

- Zinc plays an important part in glutamate regulation by exerting an inhibitory effect on NMDA receptor. Zinc is released simultaneously with glutamate during excitatory activation to regulate glutamatergic activity.[163]

- Zinc is an essential trace element shown to be deficient in migraine sufferers. The mineral plays a specific role as cofactor for adenosine deaminase production, the enzyme that breaks down adenosine.[33,34] For more information on adenosine and its prominent role in migraine pathology, refer to Chapter 2, Section 2.8, 'The role of neurotransmitters in migraine pain'.

- Zinc is also an important immune regulator an antioxidant and anti-inflammatory agent.[35] Another beneficial compound in regulating adenosine activity is the flavonoid quercetin. This antioxidant compound plays a major role in immune regulation and has shown to reduces high levels of adenosine.[36] Caffeine is also a notable inhibitor of adenosine activity and alleviates migraine headache.

Dietary sources:

Seafood (especially oysters), seaweed, red meat, chickpeas and other legumes, nuts and seeds, and dairy products.

5.7.4 Vitamin D

Prescription: Supplementary Vitamin D needs to be prescribed by a practitioner as the recommended dosage depends on the nature and severity of Vitamin D deficiency.

Administration: Oral

Instructions: Treatment needs to be monitored. It is recommended to undertake a blood test to monitor blood levels of vitamin D (calcidiol) every three months after beginning treatment. The dose may need to be adjusted based on these results to make sure normal levels are maintained.

Notes: Vitamin D is a multifunctional nutrient, essential for many pathways. The following points illustrate the vitamin's importance in migraine pathology:

- Daily doses of sunlight on your skin is the gold standard for the body to make vitamin D.

- Vitamin D stimulates the absorption of magnesium.[164]

- Vitamin D regulates brain serotonin via the expression of the *tryptophan hydroxylase 2* an enzyme that converts the amino acid *tryptophan* into serotonin.[153]

- Vitamin D promotes a *tolerogenic state* where the immune system is less likely to be overreactive or attack the body's own tissues, to preventing autoimmune diseases.[165]

- Vitamin D helps control inflammation by regulating the activity of innate immune cells, and promotes the activity of adaptive immune cells, enhancing their ability to fight infections.[165]

Caution:

- Zinc deficiency affects vitamin D activity.[166]

- Iron deficiency may impair the absorption of supplementary vitamin D and has shown to reduce hydroxylase function, which produces the active vitamin D (calcitriol).[167,168]

- Magnesium deficiency leads to lower levels of vitamin D and reduces the responsiveness of parathyroid hormone.[164]

- There are several pharmaceutical drugs that deplete vitamin D. These include laxatives. antihypertensives, antiepileptic drugs, steroids, estrogen blockers, statins,[169] and cholesterol drugs called bile acid sequestrants, which work to reduce the absorption of fats from the gut, including vitamin D.[170]

Dietary sources:

- Fatty fish (such as salmon, mackerel, trout, herring), cod liver oil, ultraviolet-treated mushrooms, and eggs.

5.8 Stress Relief Strategies and Therapies

The American philosopher William James (1842-1910) once said, 'The greatest weapon against stress is our ability to choose one thought over another.' This idea emphasises the crucial role of the mind in shaping our experiences and wellbeing. As individuals, we possess the power to choose one thought over another, significantly influencing our emotional and psychological state.

You alone have control over your stress. By choosing positive and constructive thoughts over negative or stressful ones, you can take an active role in regulating and reducing your stress levels.

Stress is not merely a response to external circumstances; it is primarily influenced by your internal thought processes and perceived stressors.

The quote underscores the importance of mindfulness and being aware of our thoughts, enabling us to consciously redirect our minds from stress-inducing thoughts to more positive and calming ones. As a mental discipline, the practice of mindfulness proactively promotes psychological resilience, which is a key strategy for combating stress.

There are three foundational strategies you can implement to strengthen your nervous system. These strategies form the groundwork, enabling your nervous system to react positively, adapt effectively and become more resilient.

- **Breathing techniques**: Implement a specific breathing method designed to help reset the nervous system, promoting calm and balance.

- **Physical activity**: Engage in regular physical activity, which triggers a natural chemical response that helps alleviate stress. This acts as both a pressure release valve and an inhibitory system to manage stress more effectively.

- **Nutritional support**: Ensure that your nervous system receives all the essential nutrients it needs to respond to stress efficiently, providing the necessary fuel for optimal function.

Now, let's delve deeper into each of these strategies to understand how they can be effectively applied to fortify your nervous system.

5.8.1 The Vagal Breathing Method

The vagal breathing method focuses on controlled breathing, also known as diaphragmatic breathing which, as you may have noticed, I have mentioned several times throughout this book. This breathing technique is not only an excellent tool for reducing stress, but it also offers a range of benefits. By improving vagal tone, it enhances lung capacity, improves oxygen saturation, reduces heart rate, and lowers blood pressure. The vagal breathing method is simple, effective and can easily be done anywhere.

When we stress, our breathing tends to become quick and shallow, a typical response indicating a state of stress or danger, which further perpetuates the stress response. Conversely, when we relax, feel at ease, or practice deep breathing exercises, it sends a signal to the brain that all is well, activating the parasympathetic nervous system. This part of the nervous system is responsible for the body's 'rest and digest' activities and helps counteract the stress response.

Deep breathing increases the supply of oxygen to the brain and stimulates the release of endorphins, which are natural mood lifters. Additionally, focusing on your breath can help distract you from stressful thoughts and promote a sense of mindfulness, which can further reduce stress levels.

The important aspect of breathing techniques is to engage your diaphragm muscles, located at the bottom of your lungs. When you inhale, instead of expanding your chest to accommodate the air, allow your belly to expand. This technique, known as belly breathing, fully engages the diaphragm muscles and maximises lung capacity. Diaphragmatic breathing stimulates the vagus nerve, which activates the parasympathetic system to take control. Regular diaphragmatic breathing improves immune function, reduced markers of chronic inflammation and oxidative stress, and regulates blood pressure.[171-173]

There are several types of vagal breathing methods, but the following technique called the 'Pursed Lip Breathing Method' is the most natural breathing technique. This method allows you to adjust to your own body and pace without the need to concentrate on counting your breaths which, unlike many other methods, can interrupt the relaxation process.

An important tip to know is that learning a breathing technique takes time and patience. At first, it may feel unfamiliar and challenging, but with regular practice, you will find it becomes easier and natural. Consistency is key. Practising the technique daily helps build muscle memory and improves control over your breath.

Pursed Lip Breathing Method

Preparation:

- Find a quiet, comfortable spot where you can either sit or lie down.

- Begin by focusing on your breathing.

- Perform a body scan: mentally move through each part of your body, asking each part to relax and release any tension.

- Return your focus to your breathing, ensuring that your inhales and exhales are deliberate and complete, but not strenuous.

- At this stage, you may feel like you're not getting enough air, which can trigger slight panic. However, this is just your mind playing tricks on you. Remind yourself that you are safe, focus on your breath, allow yourself to relax, and let your body settle into a natural rhythm.

Now that you are ready for your breathing session follow the next steps.

Breathing Session:

1. Once you are in a comfortable position, close your eyes.

2. Check for any muscle tension and relax.

3. Inhale slowly through your nose.

4. Pucker or purse your lips as if you were going to whistle.

5. Exhale slowly and gently through your pursed lips, taking longer to exhale than to inhale.

6. Repeat this process.

This should be repeated for five minutes or until you feel relaxed and calm. This exercise should be done at least twice daily. It takes a bit of practice to master and feel relaxed and calm during the exercise. Begin with one minute with the breathing exercise and gradually increase it to five minutes. Regular use of the Pursed Lip Breathing Method will improve resilience to stress, and reduce feelings of anxiety and depression. Studies have also shown that this breathing method can improve sleep[174] and promote serotonin function.[175]

I regularly use the Pursed Lip Breathing Method before I go to sleep, and in the morning before rising. You can also use an app offered by Fitbit and Apple Watch or download apps onto your phone such as *Breathe2Relax*, or *Oak-Meditation & Breathing*.

I also found the Pursed Lip Breathing Method to be the most efficient technique to stop stress induced heart palpitations. For this exercise, I recommend filling your lungs with as much air as possible and holding the inhale for 8 to 12 counts. During this interval, you will be able to feel your heartbeat and notice changes as it normalises. Slowly exhale through pursed lips until you feel there is no air left in your lungs. You may need to repeat this cycle two to five times.

Breathing Method for Heart Palpitation:

1. Inhale to fill your lungs – both belly and chest need to expand.

2. Hold for 8 to 12 counts.

3. Exhale slowly and gently through your pursed lips and feel your belly and chest fall.

4. Hold for three counts and repeat.

Repeat this process until you feel your heartbeat normalise.

5.8.2 Physical Activity

Daily physical activity is essential for maintaining good health and wellbeing. It strengthens your body and sharpens your mind. Regular exercise can enhance your mood, reduce stress and increase your energy levels, all of which are beneficial for the migraine sufferer.

Importantly, physical activity is crucial for improving lung capacity and function as well as strengthening respiratory muscles. These benefits can help reduce shallow breathing and stress-induced hypoxia. Additionally, physical activity may offer advantages for hypoxia in sleep-disordered breathing. You will find further information on these in Chapter 4, Sections 4.7 – 4.9.

Here are the following benefits:

- Improve Lung Function: Exercise can increase the efficiency of your breathing by strengthening the muscles involved in respiration, such as the diaphragm and intercostal muscles. This can help you take deeper breaths and improve the amount of oxygen that enters your lungs.

- Increase Oxygen Delivery: Regular physical activity can improve the efficiency of oxygen delivery to your muscles and brain tissue. This is achieved through improved cardiovascular function, including a stronger heart that can pump more blood per beat, and improved blood vessel function that allows for better oxygen exchange in the lungs.

- Improve Respiratory Muscle Strength: Just like any other muscle in your body, the respiratory muscles can be strengthened through regular exercise. This can improve their endurance and ability to sustain optimal function during rest and sleep.

Several studies have explored the connection between exercise and migraines, revealing that a regular routine of physical activity can reduce both the frequency and intensity of migraines.[176] This positive impact stems from the release of endorphins during physical activity. It reduces muscle tension and serves as a natural painkiller.[177] Additionally, engaging in exercise can contribute to an enhanced sense of wellbeing, setting a positive tone for the day ahead.

To make it a part of your routine, start with activities you enjoy, whether it's walking, dancing, swimming, cycling, or playing sports. Aim for at least 30 minutes of moderate exercise most days of the week. You can break this up into shorter sessions if that works better for you.

Remember, even small changes can make a big difference. Taking the stairs instead of the elevator, parking farther away and walking, or doing some stretching during TV commercials are all simple ways to add more movement to your day. The key is to find activities you love and make them a regular part of your life.

5.8.3 Feed your Stress

The title 'Feed Your Stress' might initially seem counter-intuitive but consider this: stress is a natural part of our bodily functions and a crucial survival mechanism. In this context, 'feed your stress' means providing your body with what it needs, such as a balanced diet rich in vitamins, minerals and essential nutrients to help you manage stress more effectively. It will encourage you to think differently about how to handle stress—not by avoiding or fearing it, but by fortifying your body and minds to deal with it more effectively.

Nutrients are particularly important for someone experiencing a lot of stress. When the nervous system is in chronic stress mode it can deplete certain nutrients but also increases the body's requirement for additional specific nutrients. By maintaining a diet rich in the following essential nutrients can help manage and mitigate the effects of stress.

A note of caution: While these nutrients are readily available in supplement form, their benefits are far from matching those obtained from whole foods. Supplements are man-made nutrients, typically produced in a lab or through industrial processes. These artificial nutrients are chemically similar to their natural counterparts but differ in absorption and their bioavailability.

In contrast, nutrients in whole foods work synergistically with a range of cofactors such as enzymes, fibre, flavonoids, minerals, and other vitamins within the food, creating a broader and more potent health effect that supplements simply cannot replicate.

The following list outlines the role of each essential nutrient, the effects of stress on these nutrients, and their dietary sources.

B Vitamins:

Role:

- B vitamins, particularly B6, B9 (folate), and B12, are essential for energy production, brain function and the synthesis of neurotransmitters.

Impact of Stress:

- Stress increases the body's demand for B vitamins. Deficiencies can lead to fatigue, mood disturbances and cognitive impairment.

- Dietary sources: whole grains, eggs, animal protein, and a wide variety of vegetables, especially leafy greens.

Antioxidants Vitamin E and C:

Role:

- A great antioxidant combo to combat oxidative stress in the body, which can be elevated during periods of high stress.

Important for immune function and protecting cells from oxidative damage and inflammation.

Impact of Stress:

- Stress increases oxidative stress. Insufficient antioxidant levels can lead to cellular damage and inflammatory conditions.

Dietary sources:

- Many of the following sources have a combination of vitamin E and C:

- Vitamin C: Fruit sources include berries, citrus fruits, mango, kiwi, avocado, cranberries, and olives. Vegetable sources include leafy greens, capsicum (bell peppers), cauliflower, celery, Brussels sprouts, cabbage, and broccoli.

- Vitamin E: Nuts and seeds, including almonds, hazelnuts, walnuts, hemp, sunflower seeds. This also includes plant oils such as wheat germ oil, almond oil, safflower oil, and sunflower oil (ensure they are cold-pressed and labelled as extra virgin).

Vitamin D:

Role:

- Essential for immune function and mood regulation.

- For more information on vitamin D, refer to Subsection 5.7.4

Impact of Stress:

- Low levels of vitamin D have been linked to depression and anxiety, a weakened immune response and increased susceptibility to infection and chronic disease.

Dietary sources:

- Ensuring adequate sunlight exposure for the body to make vitamin D. Fatty fish such as salmon, mackerel, trout. Fish liver oils (capsule supplements), and ultraviolet-treated mushrooms.

Magnesium:

Role:

- Magnesium helps to regulate the body's response to stress. It is involved in muscle relaxation and nerve function, and it improves electrolyte balance, energy production and sleep quality.

Impact of Stress:

- Chronic stress can deplete magnesium levels due to increased excretion in urine. Low magnesium levels may induce cortical spreading depression and increase susceptibility of vasoconstriction.

Dietary sources:

- Nuts, seeds, whole grains, dark leafy greens, avocadoes, bananas, and root vegetables like potatoes, sweet potatoes and turnips.

Zinc:

Role:

- Zinc is involved in immune function and acts as a co-factor for enzymes involved in antioxidant defence, particularly cell protection against oxidative damage. It regulates the adenosine pathway and glutamate activity.

Impact of Stress:

- Stress can reduce zinc absorption and increase its excretion. A deficiency can augment cerebral inflammation and vasodilation via increased activity of adenosine and glutamate.

Dietary sources:

- Beef, lamb, venison, shellfish, seafood, seaweed, walnuts, pecan nuts, hazelnuts, and especially Brazil nuts.

Amino Acids:

Role:

- Maintaining immune function and the production of neurotransmitters (tryptophan and tyrosine) that help regulate mood and stress. Tryptophan is essential for the production of serotonin.

Impact of Stress:

- The body requires more protein during stress to repair tissues and support immune function. Deficiencies will lead to mood disorders and increased inflammation.

Dietary sources:

- Tryptophan-rich foods include animal protein (such as beef, lamb, turkey, fish, and seafood) and eggs and cheese.

5.8.4 The Power of Quality Sleep

Good quality sleep is essential for overall health and wellbeing. There is good reason why it is called restorative sleep. During sleep, the body repairs all types of tissues, muscles, organs, blood vessels, and brain tissue. Importantly, sleep is essential for brain health. Regular good sleep builds resilience to daily stressors, regulates immune response, improves coping mechanisms, and reduces the overall perception of stress.

- **Neurotransmitter regulation**: Adequate sleep helps regulate neurotransmitter balance and reduce the risk of mood disorders such as depression and anxiety.

- **Brain plasticity**: Sleep is also critical for brain plasticity, which is the brain's ability to reorganise itself, forming new neural connections in response to learning, experience or injury. Sleep helps consolidate these new connections, supporting overall brain flexibility and adaptability.

- **Emotional regulation**: Sleep plays a role in emotional regulation, helping to process and regulate emotions. Lack of sleep can lead to increased irritability, mood swings and difficulty coping with stress.

- **Toxic clearance**: Recent research suggests that during sleep, the glymphatic system in the brain becomes more active, helping to clear away toxins and metabolic byproducts that accumulate during wakefulness. This process is thought to be important for maintaining brain health and function.

- Talk to your naturopath about natural sleep treatments.

The following sleep apps can improve sleep quality and manage sleep disorders through various methods:

Relaxation Techniques and Meditation:

- Many apps include guided relaxation exercises, breathing techniques and progressive muscle relaxation, as well as guided meditation sessions designed to reduce stress and anxiety. Some apps provide a range of soothing sounds, like white noise, nature sounds or ambient music to mask background noise and create a more conducive sleep environment. The following apps are some examples of what is available to download:

o **Calm** – This app has choice meditation tracks, relaxation music, bedtime stories, various breathing exercises, and sleep sounds.

o **Headspace** – Sleep music and soundscapes, meditation and bedtime stories,

o **Insight timer** - Gives you access to more than 80,000 soundscapes and guided meditations.

Chronic Insomnia

• Consider cognitive behavioural therapy (CBT). Ask your practitioner to help you find a CBT practitioner. Alternatively, there is an online CBT program called 'Sleepio'. https://www.sleepio.com

Some general Sleep Tips:

• Read a good novel in bed. This will take your thoughts away from the daily stressors and lull you to sleep.

• Limit Exposure to Screens Before Bed: Reduce exposure to blue light from phones, tablets, computers, and TVs at least an hour before bedtime, as it can interfere with the production of melatonin, the hormone that regulates sleep.

• Maintain a consistent sleep schedule: Go to bed and wake up at the same time every day, even on weekends, to regulate your body's internal clock.

• Create a relaxing bedtime routine: Establish a calming pre-sleep routine, such as reading, taking a warm bath, or practicing relaxation exercises, to signal your body that it's time to wind down.

- Optimise your sleep environment: Ensure your bedroom is cool, quiet and dark.

- Be mindful of your diet: Avoid large meals, sugar foods, caffeine, cordials, soft drinks, and too much alcohol close to bedtime. These can stimulate the body or cause indigestion and disrupt sleep.

- Stay active: Regular physical activity can promote better sleep. It is better to exercise earlier in the day, as working out too close to bedtime may interfere with your ability to fall asleep.

- Plenty of sunlight: Expose yourself to morning sunlight, as both sunlight and vitamin D help regulate the sleep-wake cycle.

5.9 Nitrates Strategies

If you experience frequent or chronic migraines, you may be particularly sensitive to certain triggers and nitrates may well be one of them. This is something you need to find out about personally. You may already be avoiding processed meats like ham, pastrami, bacon and such. If not, then these foods are a good gauge to identify your susceptibility to nitrates. This is where keeping a 'Migraine Diary' can be helpful. For more information on the diary, go to Chapter 5, Section 5.4. Avoiding high nitrate containing foods is a good start, and you can use the 'Trigger Foods List' (Chapter 5, Section 5.3) where you will find a comprehensive list of high nitrate foods to help you navigate this process.

Some general advice to avoid fortified nitrates in foods:

- Choose fresh foods over processed foods such as ready to eat, packaged, take out, etc.

- Read food labels carefully for both synthetic nitrate/nitrite additives and naturally occurring sources, especially in processed meats like bacon, hot dogs and deli meats. Be aware that labels claiming 'no nitrates added' may still contain naturally derived nitrates, as food industries are not required to disclose their presence.

• Organic produce and meats are less likely to contain added nitrates as organic standards restrict their use. Look for nitrate-free versions of processed meats, bacon and other foods when available.

• Cook at home. By preparing meals at home, you have more control over the ingredients and can avoid nitrate-containing additives.

Mouthwash Therapy:

1. Most of the nitrate converting bacteria are in the mouth cavity. Through regular rinsing, you can reduce the bacteria and nitrates which are generally absorbed via the salivary glands or swallowed and absorbed via the gut. The options that are available include antibacterial mouthwash (used once a day). If you would like something more natural, such as an antibacterial mouthwash, you can use warm salt water. By simply brushing your teeth regularly (after every meal) and using a water pick, you can control bacteria levels.

Alcohol:

2. Red wine has the highest nitrate content (2-20mg/L) followed by beer (1-10mg/L). It is advisable to abstain from alcohol entirely if you experience frequent or chronic migraines. As you establish a routine and become familiar with using the migraine diary and identify specific diet and lifestyle patterns, you can cautiously explore the consumption of small amounts of alcoholic beverages. You will quickly learn which beverages are better tolerated, but keep in mind that moderation is crucial as alcohol alone is a significant influential migraine trigger.

5.10 Striving for Optimal Gut Function

Optimal gut function plays a crucial role in managing and potentially preventing migraines, primarily through several interconnected pathways involving the immune system and the gut-brain axis. This axis is a complex, and still not fully understood, communication network that involves the microbiome and nervous system. Importantly, the central control system that maintains these communication pathways and metabolic processes is the gut microbiome, a microbial community that thrives in a symbiotic relationship within the gut mucosa of the host.

Poor gut health can lead to a microbial imbalance, termed 'dysbiosis', which can increase intestinal permeability (leaky gut). This condition allows pro-inflammatory substances to enter the bloodstream, leading to inflammation that can adversely impact brain function and consequently the susceptibility and sensitivity to migraine triggers.

Although the gut is a complex system of chemical interactions, maintaining a healthy gut is relatively simple. Ultimately, it is the gut bacteria that do all the work for us. All you need to do is to keep your gut bacteria well-fed.

This means providing your gut bacteria with the right nutrients and environment to thrive. Focus on a diet rich in fibre, fermented foods, polyphenols, and healthy fats and proteins, while avoiding processed foods, excess sugar and unnecessary antibiotics. Regular hydration, stress management and adequate sleep also play important roles in supporting a healthy gut microbiome.

Here are ten key points for optimal digestion and keeping your gut bacteria well-fed and thriving:

1. **Mindful Eating**

   • Mindful eating is a practice that involves paying full attention to what you eat and drink. It is about bringing awareness and intention to the experience of eating, which can lead to a greater sense of wellbeing and satisfaction with your meals. Eat slowly, chew your food thoroughly, savour each bite, and pay attention to the taste, texture and smell of your food.

- Try to avoid distractions such as TV and other electronic devices. You will find that this practice will stimulate digestion, improve nutrient absorption, and bring more awareness of your body's hunger and fullness signals.

2. Manage Your Stress

Stress can cause an unhealthy relationship with food, resulting in a negative impact on eating behaviour. This can include loss of appetite, emotional eating, overeating, or making poor food choices as a coping mechanism. In addition, this unhealthy relationship between stress and food can extend beyond eating habits and disrupt how the body processes and digests food.

During stressful moments, digestive function slows down, leading to inadequate digestion. This can result in a variety of long-term digestive issues, such as heartburn, reflux, cramping, bloating, and dysbiosis. These problems can further lead to more serious issues like food allergies, constipation, diarrhoea, irritable bowel syndrome, ulcers, and bowel cancer. Addressing your stress and practicing mindful eating habits can greatly improve digestive health.

3. Address Food Sensitivities and Triggers

Many migraine sufferers have food intolerances that can increase the sensitivity of their migraine triggers and migraine episodes. Maintaining a healthy gut can help mitigate these sensitivities and reduce the frequency of migraine triggers.

4. Avoid Overuse of Antibiotics

Antibiotics do not just eliminate harmful bacteria, but also beneficial bacteria in the gut. Therefore, it's important to take prescribed probiotics alongside a supplementary antibiotic. Also consider incorporating fermented foods into your diet to boost probiotic activity.

5. **Choose Whole Foods over Processed Foods**

Choose whole foods over processed foods. Processed foods are generally nutrient poor, high in unnecessary fats and sugars, and often contain additives and preservatives that can harm gut bacteria. In comparison, whole foods are nutrient rich and contain healthy fats, proteins, antioxidants, and fibre.

- Examples include fruits, vegetables, nuts, seeds, and animal proteins, including eggs.

6. **Dietary Fibre**

- Soluble and insoluble fibre serve as prebiotics and promote the growth and regulation of healthy gut microbes. Dietary fibre is present in all fruits and vegetables, and it is crucial to ensure that a large variety of these foods are a part of your daily diet. This is because not only fibre, but also minerals, vitamins, phytochemicals, polyphenols, and other bioactive compounds, can positively influence bacterial composition and diversity.

- Some examples of foods rich in fibre include apples, pears, bananas, broccoli, Brussels sprouts, carrots, beetroot, potatoes, nuts, legumes, and many more.

7. **Fermented Foods**

- Fermented foods are rich in probiotics, are a good source of beneficial bacteria and lactic acid to support gut health. These foods, due to their acidic nature, also stimulate digestive function by promoting the production and release of hydrochloric acid and digestive enzymes.

- Common sources of fermented foods include yogurt, kefir, sauerkraut, kimchi, miso, and kombucha.

8. Sour and Bitter Foods

- Sour and bitter foods play distinct and beneficial roles in promoting the digestive process. They induce appetite, increase saliva production, and stimulate digestive secretions, including bile, which is essential for fat digestion. This process enhances digestive efficiency and supports the breakdown and absorption of nutrients.

- Bitter foods include arugula (rocket lettuce), coffee, green tea, grapefruit, radicchio, and witlof lettuce. Common sour foods include lemon, lime, vinegar, fermented foods, pickles, rhubarb, kiwi fruit, and grapefruit.

- To optimise your digestive capacity, start your meals with a small appetizer or digestif to stimulate digestive juices. For example:

  o A small amount of apple cider vinegar or lemon juice diluted with some water. It should be no more than a tablespoon or a shot glass. Allow it to swish around the mouth for a moment before swallowing. This is also an excellent remedy for digestive complaints such as dyspepsia, bloating and heartburn.

  o A salad with a vinaigrette prior to the main meal, or some pickles to stimulate digestive juices.

- Digestif beverages after the meal can also be beneficial for digestive health.

  o **Ginger tea:** Ginger is well known for its digestive properties. Ginger tea can help alleviate nausea and stimulate digestive enzymes, enhance absorption of nutrients and reduce inflammation. A cautionary tip: ginger can be a migraine trigger for some people.

- o **Peppermint tea:** Peppermint has a soothing effect on the stomach and can help with bloating and indigestion. Consider using fresh peppermint leaves in salads and smoothies.

- o **Chamomile tea**: A soothing herbal tea that can help relax the digestive tract. It is a remarkable anti-inflammatory for digestive complaints.

- o **Fennel tea**: A tasty beverage to help reduce bloating and gas and gently stimulate digestion. Consider using fennel seeds in cooking and baking.

9. Hydration

Water is essential for hydration and plays a particularly important role in digestive function. It helps nutrient absorption, facilitates the movement of nutrients through the digestive tract, supports the activity of enzymes and other digestive compounds, and assists in the removal of waste.

The general recommendation for staying hydrated is about 3.5 litres of fluids per day for men and approximately 2.5 litres per day for woman. These are rough guidelines as hydration needs can vary, depending on several factors, including age, activity level, climate, and the type of food you eat. Whole unprocessed foods tend to contain more water than processed foods.

To stay hydrated, include fruit, vegetables and soups. Beverages like herbal teas, juices and smoothies also contribute to fluid intake. There are of course some fantastic water-rich foods like cucumbers, melons and citrus fruit.

5.10.1 Antioxidants and other Bioactive Compounds

Consuming a diet rich in the following list of antioxidants and bioactive compounds can help support a healthy gut microbiota and overall gut health.

- **Polyphenols:** Found in fruits, vegetables, tea and wine, polyphenols act as antioxidants and have anti-inflammatory properties. Examples include resveratrol, found in red wine; and quercetin, found in onions, garlic and apples, berries, grapes, and citrus fruit.

- **Flavonoids:** These are a class of polyphenols found in fruits, vegetables, tea, and red wine. Flavonoids have antioxidant and anti-inflammatory properties and promote the growth of gut bacteria.

- **Proanthocyanidins:** Found in berries, nuts and seeds. A potent antioxidant.

- **Anthocyanins:** These are a type of flavonoid found in dark blue and black fruit and vegetables, including berries, red cabbage purple sweet potatoes, red to purplish, blue-coloured leafy vegetables, and black heirloom tomatoes. Anthocyanins have antioxidant and anti-inflammatory effects.

- **Glucosinolates:** Found in cruciferous vegetables like broccoli, cabbage and kale. This compound is metabolised by gut bacteria into compounds that have anti-cancer effects and promote gut health.

- **Carotenoids:** Found in carrots, sweet potatoes spinach, and all leafy vegetables. A potent antioxidant that can benefit gut health by reducing inflammation and protecting cells.

- **Curcumin:** Found in turmeric, curcumin has antioxidant and anti-inflammatory properties.

- **Omega-3 fatty acids:** Found in fish, flaxseeds and walnuts, omega-3 fatty acids have anti-inflammatory effects that can benefit gut health by reducing inflammation in the gut and promoting the growth of beneficial bacteria.

- **Vitamin C:** Found in many fruits and vegetables, but Vitamin C is particularly high in citrus fruits, strawberries and bell peppers (capsicum). Also, kiwis, guavas and some leafy greens contain high levels of vitamin C. It is an important antioxidant that reduces oxidative stress and inflammation. As one of the bodies most effective free radical quenchers, vitamin C can support the regenerate of other antioxidant, such as vitamin E and glutathione.

- Another highly beneficial group of compounds is the thiols family. These sulfur-containing compounds offer various health benefits, including antimicrobial properties, antioxidant effects and the ability to modulate gut bacteria. The following is a list of thiols and their food sources:

- **Glutathione:** A powerful antioxidant found in many fruits, vegetables and meats. It helps reduce oxidative stress in the gut and supports the growth of beneficial bacteria.

- **Allicin:** Found in garlic and onions, allicin has antimicrobial properties that can help maintain a healthy balance of gut bacteria by inhibiting the growth of harmful bacteria.

- **Sulforaphane:** Found in cruciferous vegetables like broccoli, Brussels sprouts, bok choy, and cabbage. Sulforaphane has antioxidant and anti-inflammatory properties and overall beneficial for gut health.

- **Cysteine:** An amino acid found in high-protein foods like poultry, eggs and dairy. It is a precursor to glutathione and helps support antioxidant defences in the gut.

5.11 Optimising the Methylation Pathway

Assessing the function of the methylation pathway should be central to treatment strategies for migraines. Methylation is an essential metabolic process that occurs in most cells of the body.

In simple terms, methylation is a biochemical process that adds tiny chemical groups called methyl groups (a cluster of hydrocarbons) along DNA strands to control and regulate gene expression, producing compounds such as neurotransmitters, hormones, cell receptors, and more. This process acts like a system of checks and balances, keeping gene activity in balance by turning off certain genes when they are not needed. This ensures that genes do not become overly active or inactive, helping cells function properly.

In the context of migraines, methylation supports immune function by regulating inflammatory responses and by facilitating the synthesis and breakdown of neurotransmitters, as well as their transporters and receptors. Proper methylation ensures adequate levels and efficient metabolism of these chemicals, potentially reducing susceptibility to migraines. There are several genes involved in regulating methylation processes, and some of these genes are polymorphic. This means that they can have different genetic variants, like those found in the methylenetetrahydrofolate reductase (MTHFR) enzyme.

Each of us is different—not just on the outside, but also on the inside, with gene variations much like a fingerprint, making us all unique and contributing to what makes your body uniquely you. These genetic variants are actively functional and serve their specific roles. But like all genes, they can be influenced by epigenetics, which can directly affect gene activity. Simply put, epigenetics involve how external and internal factors such as our environment, stress, toxins, and nutrient deficiencies can impact the way genes are expressed.

The function of these genes fundamentally relies on nutrient cofactors, including specific vitamins and minerals. By providing a consistent supply of these nutrients through targeted therapeutic support, we can strengthen the related biochemical pathways and bodily systems, promoting optimal physiological function.

Methylation also plays a critical role in regulating brain function, with several factors capable of disrupting these pathways. Such disruptions can lead to either reduced activity (undermethylation) or heightened activity (overmethylation) in the production of specific biomolecules, both of which interfere with normal homeostatic balance in the brain.

To optimise the function of gene variants, it is essential to address the methylation pathway and any underlying metabolic conditions that cause inflammation and oxidative stress.

The following points highlight key factors that influence methylation and outline corresponding treatment strategies to improve brain function.

Treatment Considerations and Strategies:

- **Nutritional deficiencies** can disrupt methylation pathways, which are crucial for synthesising S-adenosylmethionine (SAMe), a primary methyl donor involved in numerous biochemical processes. Effective methylation relies on specific nutrients, including vitamins B2, B6 and B9 (folate); the minerals magnesium and zinc; and the amino acids methionine and cysteine. Insufficient levels of these nutrients can impair methylation, potentially increasing susceptibility to migraines. Tailored dietary changes, lifestyle adjustments and therapeutic approaches can improve methylation and overall health. The following strategies outline specific actions to be considered to improve methylation capacity.

- **Betaine** (Trimethylglycine) directly participates in methylation by donating methyl groups to homocysteine, thereby producing methionine and subsequently SAM. A rich source of betaine can be found in spinach, beets and whole grains such as barley, brown rice, quinoa, and especially ancient grains like spelt, emmer, rye, and khorasan. Betaine is also produced from choline within the body.

- **Choline** supports the methylation pathway by serving as a precursor to betaine and by aiding in the synthesis of phosphatidylcholine, both of which indirectly influence S-adenosylmethionine (SAM) levels. A rich source of choline is available in eggs, fish, dairy, beef, potatoes, and legumes.

- **High histamine levels** (may be associated with undermethylation). Consider supplementing with nutrients such as magnesium, zinc, methionine, inositol, vitamin B6, and vitamins A, C and E. Calcium also plays a key role in supporting undermethylation. Supplemental nutrients, including folic acid, copper, choline, and histidine may be counterproductive or potentially cause side effects in undermethylation.

- **High homocysteine** can be induced by chronic stress, resulting in nutrient depletion. This in turn increases oxidative stress and subsequently affects the function of the methylation cycle. This is because chronic stress boosts methylation demands by increasing the production of stress hormones like cortisol and adrenaline. These hormones require methylation for production and breakdown. Since homocysteine is an intermediate compound of methylation, high stress can increase its production.
Supporting homocysteine levels involves supporting the methylation pathway. Homocysteine is primarily recycled into methionine with the help of vitamin B12 and folate or converted into cysteine, which is essential for glutathione production. This process requires vitamin B6.

- **Chronic inflammation** can disrupt methylation by increasing the demand for nutrients and reducing the availability of these resources for other methylation-dependent processes.

- **Alcohol consumption** can deplete B vitamins and impair liver function, both of which are crucial for proper methylation.

- **Medication** such as antiepileptics and proton pump inhibitors, as well as frequent use of antacids, can interfere with the absorption of B vitamins and other nutrients essential for methylation.

- **Exposure to heavy metals** like lead, mercury, cadmium and arsenic can disrupt methylation by inhibiting key enzymes involved in folate metabolism. Additionally, other pollutants and chemicals, including pesticides, herbicides and various industrial compounds, can interfere with methylation processes, potentially impacting cellular function and overall health.

- **Excessive supplementation** of minerals such as calcium, iron and magnesium can disrupt folate metabolism, potentially interfering with methylation processes and adversely affecting cellular health.

- **Poor gut health**, including imbalances in the gut microbiota, can hinder the absorption of nutrients essential for methylation and produce toxins that further disrupt this pathway.

- **Detoxification** via the methylation pathways is essential for neutralising free radicals and eliminating metabolic waste products. When these detoxification processes are impaired, it can result in the accumulation of substances that trigger migraines, potentially increasing both the frequency and severity of migraine attacks.

- Inflammation and oxidative stress play key roles in the pathology of migraines. Proper methylation helps enhance antioxidant defences and regulate inflammatory responses, potentially reducing both the frequency and intensity of migraines.

Nutrient Metabolism

- Additional supportive nutrients include the sulphur-based amino acids methionine, carnitine, cysteine, and taurine. These amino acids are essential for methylation and have been found to be inadequate in the general population, particularly among individuals with insufficient animal protein in their diet.

5.12 Regulating Immune Response

The immune system plays a critical part in migraine pathology, and it is therefore vital to address any underlying imbalances and dysregulation in immunity. This can involve an overactive or underactive immune response due to conditions like allergies, frequent infections, nutrient deficiency, oxidative stress, or a broader and more severe disruption like an autoimmune condition, where there is a fundamental problem in the regulatory mechanisms that control immune responses. Reducing underlying inflammation will decrease the body's sensitivity to migraine triggers. The following subsections outline the treatment strategies for inflammatory compounds involved in this process, specifically focusing on mast cells, histamine and oxidative stress.

5.12.1 Targeting Mast Cells and Histamine

Mast cells are a type of white blood cell that play a crucial role in the immune system, particularly in the initial inflammatory process. When activated, they release various inflammatory substances, including histamine, which is a major trigger for migraines and allergic reactions. The following treatment strategies will specifically help stabilise and regulate the growth and activity of mast cells, control histamine release, and dampen allergic reactions.

Nutrients and dietary sources:

- Zinc - regulates the release of histamine.[178]

- Ascorbic acid (Vitamin C) with other bioflavonoids such as Hesperidin, Rutin and quercetin are potent mast cell inhibitor and a potent antioxidant and anti-inflammatory combo.

- Quercetin - one of the most potent mast cell stabilisers.[179]

- B6 - combined with ascorbic acid, these two vitamins synergistically work together to regulate and stabilise mast cell activity and potentiate anti-allergic properties.[180]

The flavonoids luteolin, diosmetin, myricetin, and apigenin, epigallocatechin gallate (EGCG), and quercetin, regulate mast cell activity and possess strong anti-inflammatory and antioxidant properties. The subsequent examples of fresh fruit, vegetables and herbs exhibit a significant concentration of these flavonoids.[181,182]

- Luteolin rich foods - lemons, celery, oranges, radicchio, capsicum, kohlrabi, pumpkin, chicory greens, and red leafed lettuce.

- Diosmetin rich foods - oranges, lemons, grapefruit, olives, and olive oil.

- Myricetin rich foods - cranberry, Swiss chard, rutabagas, garlic, blueberry, blackberry, peppers, and lemons.

- Apigenin rich foods - celery seeds, spinach, parsley, oregano, sage, rosemary, extra virgin vegetable oils, chamomile, and pistachio.

- Epigallocatechin gallate (EGCG) rich foods - green and black tea, berries, avocado, and some nuts, including pistachio, hazelnuts and pecans.

- Quercetin is most present in dark-coloured fruit and vegetables, and is rich in red onions, garlic, kale, broccoli, apples, berries, dark grapes, citrus fruit, and tomatoes.

Botanicals

The following medicinal plants are specific for mast cell regulation:

- Chinese Skullcap (*Scutellaria baicalensis*)[183]

- Stinging Nettle (*Urtica dioica*)[184]

- Khella Baldi (*Amni visnaga*)[185]

- Turmeric (*Curcuma longa*)[186]

- English Lavender *(Lavandula angustifolia)*

- You can also consider medicinal plants with anti-inflammatory, antioxidant, antiallergic, and adaptogenic properties to modulate immune function.

5.12.2 Inflammation and Oxidative Stress

The immune system protects the body through immune responses, commonly referred to as inflammatory responses. A healthy inflammatory response is acute, typically beneficial, and well-regulated. The body quickly mobilises immune cells to the site of injury or infection, resolving the issue promptly, and the affected tissues begin to heal.

However, when inflammation persists, the immune response remains active over a long period, continuously attempting to restore order and heal the affected tissue. Instead of protecting the body, ongoing inflammation will lead to tissue damage. Essentially, this represents a failure of the body's regulatory mechanisms, which can eventually result in autoimmune conditions and other disease states. Frequent or chronic inflammation can result from various health conditions. Below are some common examples of risk factors.

Diet and Lifestyle Factors:

Prolonged psychological stress, poor diet (leading to nutrient deficiencies), smoking, chronic alcohol consumption, and long-term exposure to irritants such as polluted air, industrial chemicals, and other toxic substances.

Infections and Autoimmune Disorders:

Persistent or frequent infections, rheumatoid arthritis, lupus, inflammatory bowel disease, psoriasis, diabetes, multiple sclerosis, and thyroid disease.

Subclinical Inflammatory Conditions:

> Common examples include obesity, blood sugar dysregulation, high blood pressure, fibromyalgia, ongoing digestive problems, and chronic allergies.

Much of the tissue damage is caused by oxidative stress, which involves an accumulation of harmful molecules known as free radicals. Under chronic stress, the production rate of free radicals increases exponentially, overwhelming the body's ability to neutralise them with antioxidants. This situation is exacerbated by a poor nutrition. Free radicals can damage cells, proteins and DNA, contributing to disease and accelerate ageing.

Frequent and chronic inflammation can result from many factors, making it crucial to find the underlying cause and implement preventive interventions to halt the progression of the inflammatory process. A general health check-up is an excellent starting point, and your naturopathic practitioner can provide you with tailored health goals to achieve this.

By following the nutrient and dietary suggestions outlined in Section 5.10 and Subsection 5.12.1, you will obtain all the anti-inflammatory and antioxidant nutrients necessary to regulate your immune system and maintain optimal antioxidant status.

5.13 Effective Treatment Strategies for Amines and Glutamate

To successfully adjust and regulate the physiological processes of amines and glutamate, you need to consider six objectives that can guide this therapeutic approach.

1st objective: Reduce the high concentrations of dietary amines and glutamate and learn to make mindful food choices. This will be your biggest challenge as you need to identify your specific food sensitivities. For this you need to use the assistance of the 'Migraine Diary' (Chapter 5, Section 5.4) and consult the 'Trigger Foods List' (Chapter 5, Section 5.3).

2nd objective: Enhancing digestive function and restoring gut bacteria (addressing dysbiosis) are key factors in regulating immune response and reducing histamine intolerance. Improving digestive function will strengthen the protective mucosal barrier, reduce inflammation, and increase the production of diamine oxidase (DAO)—the enzyme that breaks down histamine and regulates histamine production from mast cell activity. For detailed guidance on optimising your digestive health, refer to 'Striving for Optimal Gut Function' (Chapter 5, Section 5.10).

3rd objective: Evaluate the methylation pathway, which involves the production and removal of amine-degrading enzymes (DAO, HNMT, and MAO), along with their transporters and receptors. Nutrient deficiencies can impact the efficiency of this pathway. For more information, go to 'Optimising the Methylation Pathway' (Chapter 5, Section 5.11). Be mindful that optimal digestive function is essential for supporting these metabolic pathways (2nd objective).

4th objective: Assess for prescription drugs and identify any inhibitors affecting enzymatic function of DAO and MAO. Information on these pharmaceutical drugs and other factors can be found in 'The Histamine Triggers' (Chapter 3, Section 3.4) and 'The Tyramine Trigger' (Chapter 3, Section 3.5).

5th objective: Assess mast cell activity. These regulate histamine production and inflammatory responses. Focus in addressing nutrient cofactors, antioxidants and dysbiosis to achieve this goal. For more details, refer to 'Regulating Mast Cells' (Chapter 5, Section 5.12.1).

6th objective: Regulate amines by optimising enzyme function, which require specific nutrient cofactors. The following nutrients will support efficient removal of amines:

- **Vitamin B2 (flavin adenine dinucleotide (FAD))**

  o Cofactor for Monoamine oxidase (MAO) the enzyme that regulates tyramine, dopamine, norepinephrine, and serotonin.

- **Methyl group S-adenosyl-methionine (SAME)**

  o Cofactor for histamine N-methyltransferase (HNMT), responsible for breaking down histamine in every part of the body.

- **Vitamin B6, Copper (Cu) and Vitamin C**

  o diamine oxidase (DAO) responsible for breaking down histamine in the digestive tract. The combined supplementation of these nutrients has shown positive results in increased DAO activity.[187]

  o You also need to consider natural dietary sources of DAO, which are found naturally in legume sprouts, including beans, peas, chickpeas, and lentils.

  o DAO supplement, 0.3 mg per day, is common practice for histamine intolerant patients to manage their symptoms. Although supplementation can provide symptomatic relief for some, it is important to identify and address the underlying pathology of histamine intolerance for a good result.

5.14 Effective Tips for Maintaining Stable Blood Sugar Levels

Reactive hypoglycemia (low blood sugar) typically occurs between two to four hours after eating. Preventing episodes of hypoglycemia involves adopting a balanced dietary and lifestyle approach to stabilise blood sugar levels. The following is a general outline for a dietary and lifestyle protocol to help prevent reactive and fasting hypoglycemia:

Dietary Recommendations

The body needs time to adapt to a new eating regimen and to avoid any blood sugar fluctuations. It is important to eat more frequently during the day. Aim for smaller, more frequent meals every 2-4 hours. Include a balance of complex carbohydrates, quality proteins and healthy fats in each meal. These foods will help to slow down the absorption of natural sugars and are highly nutrient-dense for optimal health. Below is an example of each macronutrient:

Complex Carbohydrates:

These are high-fibre, high-nutrient dense foods, including vegetables, fruit, legumes, nuts, and whole grain, to provide a steady release of glucose.

Quality Proteins:

Protein sources such as eggs, fish, lamb, beef, chicken, seafood, and dairy products.

Healthy Fats:

Butter, olive oil, coconut oil, walnut and other nut oils, avocados, nuts, seeds. Make sure you choose oils that are cold pressed, extra virgin oils.

Avoid Sugary Foods and Highly Processed Carbohydrates:

Avoid sugary snacks, candies, soft drinks, juices, and desserts, and refined carbohydrates like white flour products, pasta and white rice as these will lead to rapid blood sugar fluctuations.

Alcoholic Beverages:

Limit alcohol intake, as it can also contribute to blood sugar imbalances.

Lifestyle Recommendations

Regular Physical Activity:

Engage in regular physical activity and exercises, including aerobic and strength training activities such as walking, running or swimming, and weightlifting or body-weight workouts. This helps to maintain stable blood sugar levels by improving muscle tone and insulin sensitivity. It also contributes to lowering stress levels.

Adequate Sleep:

Ensure you get sufficient, quality sleep each night as lack of sleep can impact insulin sensitivity and glucose metabolism.

Stress Management:

Practice stress-reducing techniques such as deep breathing, meditation or mindfulness to help manage cortisol levels and prevent stress-induced blood sugar fluctuations.

Adequate Hydration:

Drink plenty of water throughout the day to stay hydrated. Good hydration maintains optimal metabolic activity and removal of waste products.

Adequate Salt Intake:

Optimal salt intake is crucial for individuals prone to migraines. Conversely, low salt levels serve as a migraine trigger, particularly during physical activity and in warm environments, which can induce sweating. In such cases, replenishing salt levels becomes even more important to manage migraine attacks effectively.

Glossary

In alphabetical order:

Adverse effects – undesired or harmful outcome of a drug or medical treatment.
Agonist – initiates a physiological receptor response
Allele – a different form of a gene
Antagonist – inhibits a physiological receptor response
Apnoea – refers to the temporary cessation of breathing during sleep. Sleep apnea is a common condition where breathing repeatedly stops and starts during sleep
Brain plasticity or neuroplasticity is the brain's ability to change and adapt its structure and function in response to the external environment
Catalyst – a compound or substance that changes the rate of a chemical reaction
CGRP – stands for calcitonin gene-related peptide. A neuropeptide, which is a potent vasodilator and is involved in the regulation of pain and inflammation, particularly in the context of migraines
Diamine Oxidase (DAO) – enzyme that regulates histamine by breaking down the compound
Dilatation – a region of abnormal dilation
Dysbiosis is an imbalance in bacterial composition within the gut
Emesis – vomiting
Endothelium – inner wall of blood vessels. This thin layer of tissue produces compounds to maintain vasomotor changes, blood clotting factors and immune proteins
Enterocytes – cells of the intestinal lining
Ergot – a fungal disease of cereal grains such as rye.
Ergotism – poisoning by ergot, which was common in the Middle Ages when bread was made from contaminated rye flour
Exogenous – originating from an external factor, outside the body.

Extracranial – skin, muscle and blood vessels that cover surface area of the skull and facial bones.

Genotype – the genetic make-up of an individual

Homeostasis – the stable internal environment maintained by living organisms to support optimal functioning. When there is a disruption in this balance, it is due to various issues such as disease, inflammation, oxidative stress, nutrient deficiencies, or neurological disorders, depending on the nature and extent of the disturbance.

HPA axis – the hypothalamic-pituitary-adrenal axis is a mechanism that works closely with the nervous and endocrine systems by mediating the effects of stress

Hypoperfusion – inadequate blood flow to organs or tissues, often resulting in reduced oxygen and nutrient delivery

Hypopnea – overly shallow breathing or an abnormally low respiratory rate. It is often associated with sleep disorders such as sleep apnea, where a person's breathing is partially blocked or restricted during sleep, leading to reduced airflow. In the context of sleep apnoea, hypopnea refers to a decrease in airflow of at least 30% lasting for at least 10 seconds, often accompanied by a decrease in oxygen saturation in the blood

Hypoxia – the condition characterised by a deficiency of oxygen reaching the body tissues

Hypoxemia – suboptimal oxygen in the blood

Intracranial – brain and other tissue within the skull

Methylation – the methylation cycle is a biochemical pathway essential for gene expression and cell differentiation, and plays a significant role in regulating the activity of cells and metabolic systems in the body. The methylation processes in relation to migraine conditions include the nervous system, neurotransmitters, histamine and amine metabolism, liver function and its detoxification pathways, hormone regulation, and digestive health

Microbiome – refers to the community of micro-organisms (such as bacteria, viruses, fungi, and other microbes) that inhabit a particular environment. For the purposes of this book, the microbiome relates to a large community of bacteria and enzymes in the digestive tract.

Monoamine Oxidase (MAO) – enzyme that regulates amines by breaking down the compound.

Migraineur – person who suffers from migraines.

Migraine attack – the actual migraine pain period

Migraine event – the complete pathophysiological event of the migraine process from the trigger phase to the hangover phase

Neurogenic – a term used for a condition or disorder caused or controlled by, or originating in, the nervous system.

Neuromodulator – polypeptide that has the ability to potentiate or inhibit a nerve transmission

Neuropeptide – small chemical messengers produced and released by neurons for communication

Neuroplasticity, also called brain plasticity, is the brain's ability to change and adapt its structure and function in response to the external environment

Neurotransmitter – a chemical compound, also called a signalling molecule, that communicates between nerve cells (neurons) or between neurons and other target cells (like muscle cells) to facilitate communication within the nervous system. Examples include serotonin, dopamine and glutamate.

Nociception – the nervous system processing noxious stimuli that will interpret pain and an appropriate immune / defence response

Nonsteroidal Anti-Inflammatory Drugs (NSAIDs) – a class of medications that are commonly used to relieve pain, reduce inflammation and bring down a fever. Examples are Ibuprofen, Naproxen and Aspirin.

Off-target effects – signs or symptoms that can occur when a drug binds to a target other than those for which the drug was meant to bind. This can lead to unexpected side effects that may be harmful.

Peptide – a short chain of amino acids produced by the body and mostly used as chemical messengers in the nervous system

Pharmacokinetics – what the body does to the drug

Pharmacodynamics – what the drug does to the body

Pleiotropic – refers to a single factor or element that has multiple and often diverse effects or influences. This concept can apply to various fields, including genetics, biology and medicine.

Polymorphic – this is more than one variation or trait of a gene

Polypeptide – a protein molecule made up of many bonded amino acids in the formation of a chain

Premonition phase – the second phase in the migraine process. Typically relates to a feeling or perception of something that will happen. The presence of a feeling or trigger occurring prior to a migraine attack.

Receptors – specialised protein molecules on the surface of cells. They bind with specific chemical messengers such as hormones, neurotransmitters, etc, to produce a biological response.

Side effects – undesirable effects of a drug or treatment.

Subclinical condition – a health condition or disease that is not severe enough to present noticeable symptoms or clinical signs that would typically be detected during a medical examination.

Trigger phase – environmental or biochemical influences that begin the process of the migraine pathology

Vasoconstriction – the narrowing of blood vessels, particularly the arteries and arterioles, due to the contraction of the smooth muscle in their walls. This process reduces the diameter of the blood vessels, which increases vascular resistance and thereby raises blood pressure

Vasodilation – widening of blood vessels, especially the arteries and arterioles, due to the relaxation of the smooth muscle in their walls. This process increases the diameter of the blood vessels, which decreases vascular resistance and thereby lowers blood pressure

Vasomotor activity – changes in blood vessel diameter leading to either vasoconstriction or vasodilation

REFERENCES

1.   Bojazar R, Do TP, Hansen JM, Dodick DW, Ashina M. Googling migraine: A study of Google as an information resource of migraine management. *Cephalalgia.* 2020;40(14):1633-1644. doi:10.1177/0333102420942241

2.   Diener HC, Donoghue S, Gaul C, et al. Prevention of medication overuse and medication overuse headache in patients with migraine: a randomized, controlled, parallel, allocation-blinded, multicenter, prospective trial using a mobile software application. *Trials.* 2022;23(1). doi:10.1186/s13063-022-06329-2

3.   Silberstein SD. Preventive Migraine Treatment. *Contin Lifelong Learn Neurol.* 2015;21(14):613-632. doi:Silberstein S. D. (2015). Preventive Migraine Treatment. Continuum (Minneapolis, Minn.), 21(4 Headache), 973–989. https://doi.org/10.1212/CON.0000000000000199

4.   Jackson JL, Cogbill E, Santana-Davila R, et al. A comparative effectiveness meta-analysis of drugs for the prophylaxis of migraine headache. *PLoS ONE.* 2015;10(7):1-60. doi:10.1371/journal.pone.0130733

5.   Rubio-Beltrán E, Labastida-Ramírez A, Villalón CM, MaassenVanDenBrink A. Is selective 5-HT1F receptor agonism an entity apart from that of the triptans in antimigraine therapy? *Pharmacol Ther.* 2018;186:88-97. doi:10.1016/j.pharmthera.2018.01.005

6.   Pithadia A. 5-Hydroxytryptamine Receptor Subtypes and their Modulators with Therapeutic Potentials. *J Clin Med Res.* Published online 2009. doi:10.4021/JOCMR2009.05.1237

7. Leroux Andrew Buchanan Louise Lombard Li Shen Loo Daisy Bridge Ben Rousseau Natasha Hopwood Brandy Matthews Uwe Reuter ER. Evaluation of Patients with Insufficient Efficacy and/ or Tolerability to Triptans for the Acute Treatment of Migraine: A Systematic Literature Review. *Adv Ther.* 2020;37(37). doi:10.6084/m9.figshare.12902390

8. U.S. Food and Drug Administration. FAERS- adverse effect percentages of Triptans. FDA Adverse Effects Reporting System. https://fis.fda.gov/sense/app/95239e26-e0be-42d9-a960-9a5f7f1c25ee/sheet/45beeb74-30ab-46be-8267-5756582633b4/state/analysis

9. U.S. Food and Drug Administration. FAERS - Ditans. FDA Adverse Effects Reporting System. 2023. Accessed February 12, 2023. https://fis.fda.gov/sense/app/95239e26-e0be-42d9-a960-9a5f7f1c25ee/sheet/45beeb74-30ab-46be-8267-5756582633b4/state/analysis

10. Silberstein SD, Shrewsbury SB, Hoekman J. Dihydroergotamine (DHE) – Then and Now: A Narrative Review. *Headache.* 2020;60(1):40. doi:10.1111/HEAD.13700

11. Maier EF. Erfahrungen mit einer neuen Migränenbehandlung. *Med Wochenschr.* 2019;55(26):813-815. https://www.thieme.de/de/dmw-deutsche-medizinische-wochenschrift/profil-1896.htm

12. Tfelt-Hansen PC, Koehler PJ. History of the use of ergotamine and dihydroergotamine in migraine from 1906 and onward. *Cephalalgia.* 2008;28(8):877-886. doi:10.1111/J.1468-2982.2008.01578.X/ASSET/IMAGES/LARGE/10.1111_J.1468-2982.2008.01578.X-FIG2.JPEG

13. Haarmann T, Rolke Y, Giesbert S, Tudzynski P. Ergot: from witchcraft to biotechnology. Published online 2009. doi:10.1111/J.1364-3703.2009.00548.X

14. Tfelt-Hansen P, Saxena PR, Dahlöf C, et al. Ergotamine in the acute treatment of migraine. A review and European consensus. *Brain*. 2000;123(1):9-18. doi:10.1093/brain/123.1.9

15. Silberstein SD, McCrory DC. Ergotamine and Dihydroergotamine: History, Pharmacology, and Efficacy. *Headache J Head Face Pain*. 2003;43(2):144-166. doi:10.1046/j.1526-4610.2003.03034.x

16. Robbins L. New Migraine Medications: Oral Gepants, Ditan Tablet, and More. *Pract Pain Manag*. 2020;20(2). Accessed January 28, 2023. https://www.practicalpainmanagement. com/treatments/pharmacological/new-migraine-medications-oral-gepants-ditan-tablet-more

17. U.S. Food and Drug Administration. FAERS - Ergotamine Tartrate. FDA Adverse Effects Reporting System. Accessed January 28, 2023. https://fis.fda.gov/sense/app/95239e26-e0be-42d9-a960-9a5f7f1c25ee/sheet/45beeb74-30ab-46be-8267-5756582633b4/state/analysis

18. U.S. Food and Drug Administration. FAERS -Methysergide. FDA Adverse Effects Reporting System. Accessed January 28, 2023. https://fis.fda.gov/sense/app/95239e26-e0be-42d9-a960-9a5f7f1c25ee/sheet/45beeb74-30ab-46be-8267-5756582633b4/state/analysis

19. U.S. Food and Drug Administration. FAERS - adverse effect percentages -CGRP gepants and monoclonal antibody. FDA Adverse Events Reporting System. Accessed January 29, 2023. https://fis.fda.gov/sense/app/95239e26-e0be-42d9-a960-9a5f7f1c25ee/sheet/45beeb74-30ab-46be-8267-5756582633b4/state/analysis

20. Russell FA, King R, Smillie SJ, Kodji X, Brain SD. Calcitonin Gene-Related Peptide: Physiology and Pathophysiology. *Physiol Rev*. 2014;94:1099-1142. doi:10.1152/physrev.00034.2013.-Calcitonin

21. Erika Badiali SBZ Abhishek Roka. Botulinum Toxins for Headache Disorders. *Am Acad Neurol.* Published online 2021. Accessed February 14, 2023. https://www.aan.com/guidelines/home/getguidelinecontent/1169

22. Mastria G, Mancini V, Viganò A, Di Piero V. Alice in Wonderland Syndrome: A Clinical and Pathophysiological Review. *BioMed Res Int.* 2016;2016. doi:10.1155/2016/8243145

23. Mattson MP. Hormesis Defined. *Ageing Res Rev.* 2008;7(1):1-7. doi:10.1016/j.arr.2007.08.007

24. Bartsch T, Goadsby PJ. The trigeminocervical complex and migraine: Current concepts and synthesis. *Curr Pain Headache Rep.* 2003;7(5):371-376. doi:10.1007/s11916-003-0036-y

25. Ashina M, Hansen JM, Á Dunga BO, Olesen J. Human models of migraine-short-Term pain for long-Term gain. *Nat Rev Neurol.* 2017;13(12):713-724. doi:10.1038/nrneurol.2017.137

26. Jacobs B, Dussor G. Neurovascular contributions to migraine: Moving beyond vasodilation. *Neuroscience.* 2016;338:130-144. doi:10.1016/j.neuroscience.2016.06.012

27. Serotonin a la carte: Supplementation with the serotonin precursor 5-hydroxytryptophan. *Pharmacol Ther.* 2006;109(3):325-338. doi:10.1016/j.pharmthera.2005.06.004

28. Chakravarty A, Sen A. Migraine, neuropathic pain and nociceptive pain: Towards a unifying concept. *Med Hypotheses.* 2010;74(2):225-231. doi:10.1016/j.mehy.2009.08.034

29. Aggarwal M, Puri V, Puri S. Serotonin and CGRP in migraine. *Ann Neurosci.* 2012;19(2):88-94. doi:10.5214/ans.0972.7531.12190210

30. Zieglgänsberger W. Substance P and pain chronicity. *Cell Tissue Res.* 2019;375(1):227-241. doi:10.1007/s00441-018-2922-y

31. May A, Goadsby P. Substance P receptor antagonists in the therapy of migraine. *Expert Opin Investig Drugs.* 2001;10:673-678. doi:10.1517/13543784.10.4.673

32. Thuraiaiyah J, Kokoti L, Al-Karagholi MAM, Ashina M. Involvement of adenosine signaling pathway in migraine pathophysiology: a systematic review of preclinical studies. *J Headache Pain.* 2022;23(1):43. doi:10.1186/s10194-022-01412-0

33. Liu H, Wang Q, Dong Z, Yu S. Dietary zinc intake and migraine in adults: a cross-sectional analysis of the National Health and Nutrition Examination Survey 1999–2004. *Headache J Head Face Pain.* 2023;63(1):127-135. doi:10.1111/head.14431

34. Ahmadi H, Mazloumi-Kiapey SS, Sadeghi O, et al. Zinc supplementation affects favorably the frequency of migraine attacks: a double-blind randomized placebo-controlled clinical trial. *Nutr J.* 2020;19:101. doi:10.1186/s12937-020-00618-9

35. Prasad AS. Discovery of Human Zinc Deficiency: Its Impact on Human Health and Disease. *Adv Nutr.* 2013;4(2):176-190. doi:10.3945/an.112.003210

36. Atta A, Salem MM, El-Said KS, Mohamed TM. Mechanistic role of quercetin as inhibitor for adenosine deaminase enzyme in rheumatoid arthritis: systematic review. *Cell Mol Biol Lett.* 2024;29(1):14. doi:10.1186/s11658-024-00531-7

37. Pessione E, Cirrincione S. Bioactive Molecules Released in Food by Lactic Acid Bacteria: Encrypted Peptides and Biogenic Amines. *Front Microbiol.* 2016;7:876. doi:10.3389/fmicb.2016.00876

38. Fan P, Song P, Li L, Huang C, Chen J, et al. Roles of Biogenic Amines in Intestinal Signaling.pdf. *Current Protein and Peptide Science*.2017;18(6) https://pubmed. ncbi.nlm.nih.gov/27356940/#:~:text=Biogenic%20 amines%20in%20the%20gastrointestinal,%2C%20 absorption%2C%20and%20local%20immunity.

39. Sánchez-Pérez S, Comas-Basté O, Rabell-González J, Veciana-Nogués MT, Latorre-Moratalla ML, Vidal-Carou MC. Biogenic amines in plant-origin foods: Are they frequently underestimated in low-histamine diets? *Foods*. 2018;7(12). doi:10.3390/foods7120205

40. Chung BY, Park SY, Byun YS, et al. Effect of Different Cooking Methods on Histamine Levels in Selected Foods. *Ann Dermatol*. 2017;29(6):706-714. doi:10.5021/ad.2017.29.6.706

41. Pugin B, Barcik W, Westermann P, et al. A wide diversity of bacteria from the human gut produces and degrades biogenic amines. *Microb Ecol Health Dis*. 2017;28(1):1353881. doi:10.1080/16512235.2017.1353881

42. Wilkins LJ, Monga M, Miller AW. Defining Dysbiosis for a Cluster of Chronic Diseases. *Sci Rep*. 2019;9:12918. doi:10.1038/s41598-019-49452-y

43. Branco ACCC, Yoshikawa FSY, Pietrobon AJ, Sato MN. Role of Histamine in Modulating the Immune Response and Inflammation. *Mediators Inflamm*. 2018;2018. doi:10.1155/2018/9524075

44. Smolinska S, Jutel M, Crameri R, O'Mahony L. Histamine and gut mucosal immune regulation. *Allergy Eur J Allergy Clin Immunol*. 2014;69(3):273-281. doi:10.1111/all.12330

45. Mou Z, Yang Y, Hall AB, Jiang X. The taxonomic distribution of histamine-secreting bacteria in the human gut microbiome. *BMC Genomics*. 2021;22(1):695. doi:10.1186/s12864-021-08004-3

46. Sánchez-Pérez S, Comas-Basté O, Duelo A, et al. Intestinal Dysbiosis in Patients with Histamine Intolerance. *Nutrients*. 2022;14(9):1774. doi:10.3390/nu14091774

47. Schnedl WJ, Enko D. Histamine Intolerance Originates in the Gut. *Nutrients*. 2021;13(4):1262. doi:10.3390/nu13041262

48. Meza-Velázquez R, López-Márquez F, Espinosa-Padilla S, Rivera-Guillen M, Ávila-Hernández J, Rosales-González M. Association of diamine oxidase and histamine N-methyltransferase polymorphisms with presence of migraine in a group of Mexican mothers of children with allergies. *Neurol Engl Ed*. 2017;32(8):500-507. doi:10.1016/j.nrleng.2016.02.012

49. Worm J, Falkenberg K, Olesen J. Histamine and migraine revisited: Mechanisms and possible drug targets. *J Headache Pain*. 2019;20(1):1-12. doi:10.1186/s10194-019-0984-1

50. Yuan H, Silberstein SD. Histamine and Migraine. *Headache*. 2018;58(1):184-193. doi:10.1111/head.13164

51. Alstadhaug KB. Histamine in Migraine and Brain. *Headache J Head Face Pain*. 2014;54(2):246-259. doi:10.1111/head.12293

52. Millán-Guerrero RO, Baltazar-Rodríguez LM, Cárdenas-Rojas MI, et al. A280V Polymorphism in the Histamine H3 Receptor as a Risk Factor for Migraine. *Arch Med Res*. 2011;42(1):44-47. doi:10.1016/j.arcmed.2011.01.009

53. Corazza GR, Falasca A, Strocchi A, Rossi CA, Gasbarrini G. Decreased plasma postheparin diamine oxidase levels in celiac disease. *Dig Dis Sci*. 1988;33(8):956-961. doi:10.1007/BF01535991

54. Leitner R, Zoernpfenning E, Missbichler A. Evaluation of the inhibitory effect of various drugs / active ingredients on the activity of human diamine oxidase in vitro. *Clin Transl Allergy.* 2014;4(Suppl 3):P23. doi:10.1186/2045-7022-4-S3-P23

55. Burns C, Kidron A. Biochemistry, Tyramine. In: *StatPearls.* StatPearls Publishing; 2023. Accessed July 23, 2023. http://www.ncbi.nlm.nih.gov/books/NBK563197/

56. Koh AHW, Chess-Williams R, Lohning AE. Differential mechanisms of action of the trace amines octopamine, synephrine and tyramine on the porcine coronary and mesenteric artery. *Sci Rep.* 2019;9(1). doi:10.1038/s41598-019-46627-5

57. D'Andrea G, D'Amico D, Bussone G, et al. The role of tyrosine metabolism in the pathogenesis of chronic migraine. *Cephalalgia Int J Headache.* 2013;33(11):932-937. doi:10.1177/0333102413480755

58. Sved AF, Weeks JJ, Grace AA, Smith TT, Donny EC. Monoamine oxidase inhibition in cigarette smokers: From preclinical studies to tobacco product regulation. *Front Neurosci.* 2022;16:886496. doi:10.3389/fnins.2022.886496

59. Rafehi M, Faltraco F, Matthaei J, et al. Highly Variable Pharmacokinetics of Tyramine in Humans and Polymorphisms in OCT1, CYP2D6, and MAO-A. *Front Pharmacol.* 2019;10:1297. doi:10.3389/fphar.2019.01297

60. Shumay E, Logan J, Volkow ND, Fowler JS. Evidence that the methylation state of the monoamine oxidase A (MAOA) gene predicts brain activity of MAOA enzyme in healthy men. *Epigenetics.* 2012;7(10):1151-1160. doi:10.4161/epi.21976

61. Hawkins RA. The blood-brain barrier and glutamate1234. *Am J Clin Nutr.* 2009;90(3):867S-874S. doi:10.3945/ajcn.2009.27462BB

62. Park CG, Chu MK. Interictal plasma glutamate levels are elevated in individuals with episodic and chronic migraine. *Nat Portf.* 2022;(12). doi:10.1038/s41598-022-10883-9

63. Benbow T, Cairns BE. Dysregulation of the peripheral glutamatergic system: A key player in migraine pathogenesis? *Cephalalgia.* 2021;41(11-12):1249-1261. doi:10.1177/03331024211017882

64. Benbow T, Cairns BE. Dysregulation of the peripheral glutamatergic system: A key player in migraine pathogenesis? doi:10.1177/03331024211017882

65. Nutr A, Loï C, Cynober L. Human Nutrition: Review Article Glutamate: A Safe Nutrient, Not Just a Simple Additive. Published online 2017. doi:10.1159/000522482

66. Umami Information Center. 2023. Accessed April 2, 2023. https://www.umamiinfo.com/

67. Amin Z, Canli T, Epperson CN. Effect of estrogen-serotonin interactions on mood and cognition. *Behav Cogn Neurosci Rev.* 2005;4(1):43-58. doi:10.1177/1534582305277152

68. Barth C, Villringer A, Sacher J. Sex hormones affect neurotransmitters and shape the adult female brain during hormonal transition periods. *Front Neurosci.* 2015;9:37. doi:10.3389/fnins.2015.00037

69. Borkum JM. Migraine Triggers and Oxidative Stress: A Narrative Review and Synthesis. *Headache J Head Face Pain.* 2016;56(1):12-35. doi:10.1111/head.12725

70. Gudipally PR, Sharma GK. Premenstrual Syndrome. In: *StatPearls.* StatPearls Publishing; 2023. Accessed November 23, 2023. http://www.ncbi.nlm.nih.gov/books/NBK560698/

71. Aggarwal M, Puri V, Puri S. Serotonin and CGRP in Migraine. *Ann Neurosci.* 2012;19(2):88-94. doi:10.5214/ans.0972.7531.12190210

72. Del Moro L, Rota E, Pirovano E, Rainero I. Migraine, Brain Glucose Metabolism and the "Neuroenergetic" Hypothesis: A Scoping Review. *J Pain.* 2022;23(8):1294-1317. doi:10.1016/j.jpain.2022.02.006

73. Stress, hypoglycemia, and the autonomic nervous system. *Auton Neurosci.* 2022;240:102983. doi:10.1016/j.autneu.2022.102983

74. Gallai V, Alberti A, Gallai B, Coppola F, Floridi A, Sarchielli P. Glutamate and Nitric Oxide Pathway in Chronic Daily Headache: Evidence From Cerebrospinal Fluid. *Cephalalgia.* 2003;23(3):166-174. doi:10.1046/j.1468-2982.2003.00552.x

75. Henderson W, Raskin N. "HOT-DOG" HEADACHE: INDIVIDUAL SUSCEPTIBILITY TO NITRITE. *The Lancet.* 1972;300(7788):1162-1163. doi:10.1016/S0140-6736(72)92591-3

76. Hord NG, Tang Y, Bryan NS. Food sources of nitrates and nitrites: the physiologic context for potential health benefits2. *Am J Clin Nutr.* 2009;90(1):1-10. doi:10.3945/ajcn.2008.27131

77. Silva-Néto RP, de Almeida Soares A, Augusto Carvalho de Vasconcelos C, da Silva Lopes L. Watermelon and others plant foods that trigger headache in migraine patients. *Postgrad Med.* 2021;133(7):760-764. doi:10.1080/00325481.2021.1922211

78. Silva-Néto RP, Bezerra GL, Araújo NRA, et al. Migraine Attacks Triggered by Ingestion of Watermelon. *Eur Neurol.* 2023;86(4):250-255. doi:10.1159/000531286

79. Cosby K, Partovi KS, Crawford JH, et al. Nitrite reduction to nitric oxide by deoxyhemoglobin vasodilates the human circulation. *Nat Med.* 2003;9(12):1498-1505. doi:10.1038/nm954

80. Thomsen L l., Kruuse C, Iversen H k., Olesen J. A nitric oxide donor (nitroglycerin) triggers genuine migraine attacks. *Eur J Neurol.* 1994;1(1):73-80. doi:10.1111/j.1468-1331.1994.tb00053.x

81. Iversen HK, Olesen J, Tfelt-Hansen P. Intravenous nitroglycerin as an experimental model of vascular headache. Basic characteristics. *Pain.* 1989;38(1):17-24. doi:10.1016/0304-3959(89)90067-5

82. Olesen J, Iversen HK, Thomsen LL. Nitric oxide supersensitivity: a possible molecular mechanism of migraine pain. *NeuroReport.* 1993;4(8):1027. doi.org/10.1097/00001756-199308000-00008

83. Neyal M, Geyik S, Cekmen M, Balat A, Neyal A. Elevated plasma total nitrite levels may be related to migraine attacks. *Gaziantep Med J.* 2014;20:299. doi:10.5455/GMJ-30-160373

84. Lidder S, Webb AJ. Vascular effects of dietary nitrate (as found in green leafy vegetables and beetroot) via the nitrate-nitrite-nitric oxide pathway. *Br J Clin Pharmacol.* 2013;75(3):677-696. doi:10.1111/j.1365-2125.2012.04420.x

85. Sweazea KL, Johnston CS, Miller B, Gumpricht E. Nitrate-Rich Fruit and Vegetable Supplement Reduces Blood Pressure in Normotensive Healthy Young Males without Significantly Altering Flow-Mediated Vasodilation: A Randomized, Double-Blinded, Controlled Trial. *J Nutr Metab.* 2018;2018:1729653. doi:10.1155/2018/1729653

86. Bondonno CP, Liu AH, Croft KD, et al. Antibacterial mouthwash blunts oral nitrate reduction and increases blood pressure in treated hypertensive men and women. *Am J Hypertens.* 2015;28(5):572-575. doi:10.1093/ajh/hpu192

87. Gonzalez A, Hyde E, Sangwan N, Gilbert JA, Viirre E, Knight R. Migraines Are Correlated with Higher Levels of Nitrate-, Nitrite-, and Nitric Oxide-Reducing Oral Microbes in the American Gut Project Cohort. *mSystems*. 2016;1(5):10.1128/msystems.00105-16. doi:10.1128/msystems.00105-16

88. González-Soltero R, Bailén M, de Lucas B, Ramírez-Goercke MI, Pareja-Galeano H, Larrosa M. Role of Oral and Gut Microbiota in Dietary Nitrate Metabolism and Its Impact on Sports Performance. *Nutrients*. 2020;12(12):3611. doi:10.3390/nu12123611

89. Govoni M, Jansson EÅ, Weitzberg E, Lundberg JO. The increase in plasma nitrite after a dietary nitrate load is markedly attenuated by an antibacterial mouthwash. *Nitric Oxide*. 2008;19(4):333-337. doi:10.1016/j.niox.2008.08.003

90. Toda N, Ayajiki K. Vascular Actions of Nitric Oxide as Affected by Exposure to Alcohol. *Alcohol Alcohol*. 2010;45(4):347-355. doi:10.1093/alcalc/agq028

91. Gazzieri D, Trevisani M, Tarantini F, et al. Ethanol dilates coronary arteries and increases coronary flow via transient receptor potential vanilloid 1 and calcitonin gene-related peptide. *Cardiovasc Res*. 2006;70(3):589-599. doi:10.1016/j.cardiores.2006.02.027

92. Deng X sheng, Deitrich RA. Ethanol Metabolism and Effects: Nitric Oxide and its Interaction. *Curr Clin Pharmacol*. 2007;2(2):145-153. doi:10.2174/157488407780598135

93. Panconesi A. Serotonin and migraine: a reconsideration of the central theory. *J Headache Pain*. 2008;9(5):267-276. doi:10.1007/s10194-008-0058-2

94. Dreiseitel A, Korte G, Schreier P, et al. Berry anthocyanins and their aglycons inhibit monoamine oxidases A and B. *Pharmacol Res*. 2009;59(5):306-311. doi:10.1016/j.phrs.2009.01.014

95. Zivadinov R, Willheim K, Sepic-Grahovac D, et al. Migraine and tension-type headache in Croatia: a population-based survey of precipitating factors. *Cephalalgia Int J Headache.* 2003;23(5):336-343. doi:10.1046/j.1468-2982.2003.00544.x

96. Peatfield RC. Relationships between food, wine, and beer-precipitated migrainous headaches. *Headache.* 1995;35(6):355-357. doi:10.1111/j.1526-4610.1995.hed3506355.x

97. Spierings ELH, Ranke AH, Honkoop PC. Precipitating and Aggravating Factors of Migraine Versus Tension-type Headache. *Headache J Head Face Pain.* 2001;41(6):554-558. doi:10.1046/j.1526-4610.2001.041006554.x

98. Fried NT, Elliott MB, Oshinsky ML. The Role of Adenosine Signaling in Headache: A Review. *Brain Sci.* 2017;7(3):30. doi:10.3390/brainsci7030030

99. Deus VL, Bispo ES, Franca AS, Gloria MBA. Understanding amino acids and bioactive amines changes during on-farm cocoa fermentation. *J Food Compos Anal.* 2021;97:103776. doi:10.1016/j.jfca.2020.103776

100. Nowaczewska M, Wiciński M, Kaźmierczak W, Kaźmierczak H. To Eat or Not to eat: A Review of the Relationship between Chocolate and Migraines. *Nutrients.* 2020;12(3):608. doi:10.3390/nu12030608

101. van den Bogaard B, Draijer R, Westerhof BE, van den Meiracker AH, van Montfrans GA, van den Born BJH. Effects on Peripheral and Central Blood Pressure of Cocoa With Natural or High-Dose Theobromine. *Hypertension.* 2010;56(5):839-846. doi:10.1161/hypertensionaha.110.158139

102. Zugravu C, Otelea MR. Dark Chocolate: To Eat or Not to Eat? A Review. *J AOAC Int.* 2019;102(5):1388-1396. doi:10.1093/jaoac/102.5.1388

103. Chen M, Yan HH, Shu S, et al. Amygdalar Endothelin-1 Regulates Pyramidal Neuron Excitability and Affects Anxiety. *Sci Rep*. 2017;7(1):1-14. doi:10.1038/s41598-017-02583-6

104. Edvinsson L, Haanes KA, Warfvinge K. Does inflammation have a role in migraine? *Nat Rev Neurol*. 2019;15(8):483-490. doi:10.1038/s41582-019-0216-y

105. Liu YZ, Wang YX, Jiang CL. Inflammation: The Common Pathway of Stress-Related Diseases. *Front Hum Neurosci*. 2017;11:316. doi:10.3389/fnhum.2017.00316

106. Mcewen BS, Bowles NP, Gray JD, et al. Mechanisms of stress in the brain. doi:10.1038/nn.4086

107. Arnsten AFT, Raskind MA, Taylor FB, Connor DF. The effects of stress exposure on prefrontal cortex: Translating basic research into successful treatments for post-traumatic stress disorder. *Neurobiol Stress*. 2015;1(1):89-99. doi:10.1016/J.YNSTR.2014.10.002

108. Arnsten AFT. Stress signalling pathways that impair prefrontal cortex structure and function. Published online 2009. doi:10.1038/nrn2648

109. McEwen BS. Physiology and neurobiology of stress and adaptation: Central role of the brain. *Physiol Rev*. 2007;87(3):873-904. doi:10.1152/PHYSREV.00041.2006/ASSET/IMAGES/LARGE/Z9J0030724460008.JPEG

110. Negm M, Housseini AM, Abdelfatah M, Asran A. Relation between migraine pattern and white matter hyperintensities in brain magnetic resonance imaging. doi:10.1186/s41983-018-0027-x

111. Bashir A, Lipton RB, Ashina S, Ashina M. *VIEWS & REVIEWS Migraine and Structural Changes in the Brain A Systematic*

Review and Meta-Analysis.; 2013. Accessed December 28, 2022. https://www.ncbi.nlm.nih.gov/pmc/articles/PMC3795609/

112. Habes M, Sotiras A, Erus G, et al. White matter lesions Spatial heterogeneity, links to risk factors, cognition, genetics, and atrophy. *Neurol ®.* 2018;91:964-975. doi:10.1212/WNL.0000000000006116

113. Chen Y, Xu J, Chen Y. Regulation of Neurotransmitters by the Gut Microbiota and Effects on Cognition in Neurological Disorders. *Nutrients.* 2021;13(6):2099. doi:10.3390/nu13062099

114. Aurora SK, Shrewsbury SB, Ray S, Hindiyeh N, Nguyen L. A link between gastrointestinal disorders and migraine: Insights into the gut–brain connection. *Headache J Head Face Pain.* 2021;61(4):576-589. doi:10.1111/head.14099

115. Burnouf T, Walker TL. The multifaceted role of platelets in mediating brain function. *Blood.* 2022;140(8):815-827. doi:10.1182/blood.2022015970

116. De Deurwaerdère P, Di Giovanni G. Serotonin in Health and Disease. *Int J Mol Sci.* 2020;21(10):3500. doi:10.3390/ijms21103500

117. G E Tafet VPIV DP Abulafia, JM Calandria, SS Roffman, A Chiovetta, M Shinitzky. Correlation between cortisol level and serotonin uptake in patients with chronic stress and depression. *Cogn Affect Behav Neurosci.* 2001;1(4):388-393. DOI: 10.3758/cabn.1.4.388

118. Woldeamanuel YW, Sanjanwala BM, Cowan RP. Endogenous glucocorticoids may serve as biomarkers for migraine chronification. *Ther Adv Chronic Dis.* 2020;11:2040622320939793. doi:10.1177/2040622320939793

119. Badawy AAB, Dawood S, Bano S. Kynurenine pathway of tryptophan metabolism in pathophysiology and therapy of major depressive disorder. *World J Psychiatry*. 2023;13(4):141-148. doi:10.5498/wjp.v13.i4.141

120. MD CW. Evaluating Cerebral Blood Flow Velocity During Migraine Headache. Neurology Advisor. 2017. Accessed December 21, 2023. https://www.neurologyadvisor. com/topics/migraine-and-headache/evaluating-cerebral-blood-flow-velocity-during-migraine-headache/

121. Denuelle M, Fabre N, Payoux P, Chollet F, Geraud G. Posterior cerebral hypoperfusion in migraine without aura. *Cephalalgia Int J Headache*. 2008;28(8):856-862. doi:10.1111/j.1468-2982.2008.01623.x

122. Fu T, Liu L, Huang X, et al. Cerebral blood flow alterations in migraine patients with and without aura: An arterial spin labeling study. *J Headache Pain*. 2022;23(1):131. doi:10.1186/s10194-022-01501-0

123. Olesen J, Friberg L, Olsen TS, et al. Timing and topography of cerebral blood flow, aura, and headache during migraine attacks. *Ann Neurol*. 1990;28(6):791-798. doi:10.1002/ana.410280610

124. Mason BN, Russo AF. Vascular contributions to migraine: Time to revisit? *Front Cell Neurosci*. 2018;12:233. doi:10.3389/FNCEL.2018.00233/BIBTEX

125. Iljazi A, Ayata C, Ashina M, Hougaard A. The Role of Endothelin in the Pathophysiology of Migraine—a Systematic Review. *Curr Pain Headache Rep*. 2018;22(4). doi:10.1007/s11916-018-0682-8

126. Fox BM, Becker BK, Loria AS, et al. Acute pressor response to psychosocial stress is dependent on endothelium-derived endothelin-1. *J Am Heart Assoc*. 2018;7(4). doi:10.1161/JAHA.117.007863

127. Schoenen J. Hypoxia, a turning point in migraine pathogenesis? *Brain.* 2016;139(3):644-647. doi:10.1093/brain/awv402

128. Frank F, Kaltseis K, Filippi V, Broessner G. Hypoxia-related mechanisms inducing acute mountain sickness and migraine. *Front Physiol.* 2022;13. Accessed December 2, 2023. https://www.frontiersin.org/articles/10.3389/fphys.2022.994469

129. Burtscher M, Hefti U, Hefti JP. High-altitude illnesses: Old stories and new insights into the pathophysiology, treatment and prevention. *Sports Med Health Sci.* 2021;3(2):59-69. doi:10.1016/j.smhs.2021.04.001

130. Linde M, Edvinsson L, Manandhar K, Risal A, Steiner TJ. Migraine associated with altitude: results from a population-based study in Nepal. *Eur J Neurol.* 2017;24(8):1055-1061. doi:10.1111/ene.13334

131. Arregui A, Cabrera J, Leon-Velarde F, Paredes S, Viscarra D, Arbaiza D. High prevalence of migraine in a high-altitude population. *Neurology.* 1991;41(10):1668-1669. doi:10.1212/wnl.41.10.1668

132. Manandhar K, Risal A, Steiner TJ, Holen A, Linde M. The prevalence of primary headache disorders in Nepal: a nationwide population-based study. *J Headache Pain.* 2015;16:95. doi:10.1186/s10194-015-0580-y

133. Mojadidi MK, Ruiz JC, Chertoff J, et al. Patent Foramen Ovale and Hypoxemia. *Cardiol Rev.* 2019;27(1):34-40. doi:10.1097/CRD.0000000000000205

134. Wang M, Lan D, Dandu C, Ding Y, Ji X, Meng R. Normobaric oxygen may attenuate the headache in patients with patent foramen povale and migraine. *BMC Neurol.* 2023;23(1):44. doi:10.1186/s12883-023-03059-z

135. Zhang Y, Wang H, Liu L. Patent Foramen Ovale Closure for Treating Migraine: A Meta-Analysis. *J Intervent Cardiol.* 2022;2022:6456272. doi:10.1155/2022/6456272

136. Chaliha DR, Vaccarezza M, Takechi R, et al. A paradoxical vasodilatory nutraceutical intervention for prevention and attenuation of migraine—a hypothetical review. *Nutrients.* 2020;12(8):1-15. doi:10.3390/nu12082487

137. Fried NT, Elliott MB, Oshinsky ML. The role of adenosine signaling in headache: A review. *Brain Sci.* 2017;7(3). doi:10.3390/brainsci7030030

138. Wang Y, Wang Y, Yue G, Zhao Y. Energy metabolism disturbance in migraine: From a mitochondrial point of view. *Front Physiol.* 2023;14:1133528. doi:10.3389/fphys.2023.1133528

139. Brzecka A. Role of hypercapnia in brain oxygenation in sleep-disordered breathing. *Acta Neurobiol Exp (Warsz).* 2007;67(2):197-206. https://pubmed.ncbi.nlm.nih.gov/17691228/

140. Schoenen J. Hypoxia, a turning point in migraine pathogenesis? *Brain.* 2016;139(3):644-647. doi:10.1093/BRAIN/AWV402

141. Santilli M, Manciocchi E, D'Addazio G, et al. Prevalence of Obstructive Sleep Apnea Syndrome: A Single-Center Retrospective Study. *Int J Environ Res Public Health.* 2021;18(19):10277. doi:10.3390/ijerph181910277

142. Won L, Nagubadi S, Kryger MH, Mokhlesi B. Epidemiology of Obstructive Sleep Apnea: a Population-based Perspective. *Expert Rev Respir Med.* 2008;2(3):349. doi:10.1586/17476348.2.3.349

143. Mariotti Agnese. The effects of chronic stress on health: new insights into the molecular mechanisms of brain–body communication. Published online 2015. doi:10.4155/FSO.15.21

144. Won CHJ, Qin L, Selim B, Yaggi HK. Varying hypopnea definitions affect obstructive sleep apnea severity classification and association with cardiovascular disease. *J Clin Sleep Med*. 2018;14(12):1987-1994. doi:10.5664/jcsm.7520

145. Frangopoulos F, Zannetos S, Nicolaou I, et al. The Complex Interaction Between the Major Sleep Symptoms, the Severity of Obstructive Sleep Apnea, and Sleep Quality. *Front Psychiatry*. 2021;12:155. doi:10.3389/FPSYT.2021.630162/BIBTEX

146. Baker-Smith CM, Isaiah A, Melendres MC, et al. Sleep-Disordered Breathing and Cardiovascular Disease in Children and Adolescents: A Scientific Statement From the American Heart Association. *J Am Heart Assoc Cardiovasc Cerebrovasc Dis*. 2021;10(18):22427. doi:10.1161/JAHA.121.022427

147. Douglas NJ, White DP, Pickett CK, Weil JV, Zwillich CW. Respiration during sleep in normal man. *Thorax*. 1982;37(11):840-844. https://www.ncbi.nlm.nih.gov/pmc/articles/PMC459437/

148. Siegel JM. The Neurotransmitters of Sleep. *J Clin Psychiatry*. 2004;65(16):4-7. https://www.ncbi.nlm.nih.gov/pmc/articles/PMC8761080/

149. Lambert G, Reid C, Kaye D, Jennings G, Esler M. Effect of sunlight and season on serotonin turnover in the brain. *The Lancet*. 2002;360(9348):1840-1842. doi:10.1016/S0140-6736(02)11737-5

150. Sansone RA, Sansone LA. Sunshine, Serotonin, and Skin: A Partial Explanation for Seasonal Patterns in Psychopathology? *Innov Clin Neurosci*. 2013;10(7-8):20. https://pmc.ncbi.nlm.nih.gov/articles/PMC3779905/

151. Portas CM, Bjorvatn B, Ursin R. Serotonin and the sleep/wake cycle: special emphasis on microdialysis studies. *Prog Neurobiol.* 2000;60(1):13-35. doi:10.1016/S0301-0082(98)00097-5

152. Melrose S. Seasonal Affective Disorder: An Overview of Assessment and Treatment Approaches. *Depress Res Treat.* 2015;2015:178564. doi:10.1155/2015/178564

153. Huiberts LM, Smolders KCHJ. Effects of vitamin D on mood and sleep in the healthy population: Interpretations from the serotonergic pathway. *Sleep Med Rev.* 2021;55:101379. doi:10.1016/j.smrv.2020.101379

154. Maes M, Van Gastel A, Ranjan R, et al. Stimulatory effects of L-5-hydroxytryptophan on postdexamethasone beta-endorphin levels in major depression. *Neuropsychopharmacol Off Publ Am Coll Neuropsychopharmacol.* 1996;15(4):340-348. doi:10.1016/0893-133X(95)00238-9

155. Aliño JJ, Gutierrez JL, Iglesias ML. 5-Hydroxytryptophan (5-HTP) and a MAOI (nialamide) in the treatment of depressions. A double-blind controlled study. *Int Pharmacopsychiatry.* 1976;11(1):8-15. doi:10.1159/000468207

156. Nicolodi M, Sicuteri F. Fibromyalgia and migraine, two faces of the same mechanism. Serotonin as the common clue for pathogenesis and therapy. *Adv Exp Med Biol.* 1996;398:373-379. doi:10.1007/978-1-4613-0381-7_58

157. Cummings JL. Alternatives to Psychotherapy. In: Hersen M, Sledge W, eds. *Encyclopedia of Psychotherapy.* Academic Press; 2002:33-40. doi:10.1016/B0-12-343010-0/00005-2

158. Na HS, Ryu JH, Do SH. The role of magnesium in pain. In: Vink R, Nechifor M, eds. *Magnesium in the Central Nervous System.* University of Adelaide Press; 2011. Accessed June 12, 2024. http://www.ncbi.nlm.nih.gov/books/NBK507245/

159. Guerrero-Toro C, Koroleva K, Ermakova E, et al. Citation: Testing the Role of Glutamate NMDA Receptors in Peripheral Trigeminal Nociception Implicated in Migraine Pain. Published online 2022. doi:10.3390/ijms23031529

160. Maier JAM, Locatelli L, Fedele G, Cazzaniga A, Mazur A. Magnesium and the Brain: A Focus on Neuroinflammation and Neurodegeneration. *Int J Mol Sci.* 2023;24(1):223. doi:10.3390/ijms24010223

161. Mathew AA, Panonnummal R. 'Magnesium'-the master cation-as a drug—possibilities and evidences. *BioMetals.* 2021;34(5):955-986. doi:10.1007/s10534-021-00328-7

162. Schwalfenberg GK, Genuis SJ. The Importance of Magnesium in Clinical Healthcare. *Scientifica.* 2017;2017:4179326. doi:10.1155/2017/4179326

163. Granzotto A, Canzoniero LMT, Sensi SL. A Neurotoxic Ménage-à-trois: Glutamate, Calcium, and Zinc in the Excitotoxic Cascade. *Front Mol Neurosci.* 2020;13. doi:10.3389/fnmol.2020.600089

164. Uwitonze AM, Razzaque MS. Role of Magnesium in Vitamin D Activation and Function. *J Osteopath Med.* 2018;118(3):181-189. doi:10.7556/jaoa.2018.037

165. Ghaseminejad-Raeini A, Ghaderi A, Sharafi A, et al. Immunomodulatory actions of vitamin D in various immune-related disorders: a comprehensive review. *Front Immunol.* 2023;14. doi:10.3389/fimmu.2023.950465

166. Amos A, Razzaque MS. Zinc and its role in vitamin D function. *Curr Res Physiol.* 2022;5:203. doi:10.1016/j.crphys.2022.04.001

167. Azizi-Soleiman F, Vafa M, Abiri B, Safavi M. Effects of Iron on Vitamin D Metabolism: A Systematic Review. *Int J Prev Med.* 2016;7:126. doi:10.4103/2008-7802.195212

168. Mogire RM, Muriuki JM, Morovat A, et al. Vitamin D Deficiency and Its Association with Iron Deficiency in African Children. *Nutrients*. 2022;14(7):1372. doi:10.3390/nu14071372

169. Gröber U, Kisters K. Influence of drugs on vitamin D and calcium metabolism. *Dermatoendocrinol*. 2012;4(2):158. doi:10.4161/derm.20731

170. Hameed MH, Patel P, Farzam K. Colestipol. In: *StatPearls*. StatPearls Publishing; 2024. Accessed November 2, 2024. http://www.ncbi.nlm.nih.gov/books/NBK587349/

171. Li T ting, Wang H ying, Zhang H, et al. Effect of breathing exercises on oxidative stress biomarkers in humans: A systematic review and meta-analysis. *Front Med*. 2023;10:1121036. doi:10.3389/fmed.2023.1121036

172. Wang CH, Yang HW, Huang HL, et al. Long-Term Effect of Device-Guided Slow Breathing on Blood Pressure Regulation and Chronic Inflammation in Patients with Essential Hypertension Using a Wearable ECG Device. *Acta Cardiol Sin*. 2021;37(2):195-203. doi:10.6515/ACS.202103_37(2).20200907A

173. Russo MA, Santarelli DM, O'Rourke D. The physiological effects of slow breathing in the healthy human. *Breathe*. 2017;13(4):298-309. doi:10.1183/20734735.009817

174. Jerath R, Beveridge C, Barnes VA. Self-Regulation of Breathing as an Adjunctive Treatment of Insomnia. *Front Psychiatry*. 2018;9(JAN). doi:10.3389/FPSYT.2018.00780

175. Hilaire G, Voituron N, Menuet C, Ichiyama RM, Subramanian HH, Dutschmann M. THE ROLE OF SEROTONIN IN RESPIRATORY FUNCTION AND DYSFUNCTION. *Respir Physiol Neurobiol*. 2010;174(1-2):76-88. doi:10.1016/j.resp.2010.08.017

176. Amin FM, Aristeidou S, Baraldi C, et al. The association between migraine and physical exercise. *J Headache Pain.* 2018;19(1):83. doi:10.1186/s10194-018-0902-y

177. Ahn AH. Why does increased exercise decrease migraine? *Curr Pain Headache Rep.* 2013;17(12):379. doi:10.1007/s11916-013-0379-y

178. Nishida K, Uchida R. Role of Zinc Signaling in the Regulation of Mast Cell-, Basophil-, and T Cell-Mediated Allergic Responses. *J Immunol Res.* 2018;2018:5749120. doi:10.1155/2018/5749120

179. Theoharides TC, Donelan J, Kandere-Grzybowska K, Konstantinidou A. The role of mast cells in migraine pathophysiology. *Brain Res Rev.* 2005;49(1):65-76. doi:10.1016/j.brainresrev.2004.11.006

180. Kazama I, Sato Y, Tamada T. Pyridoxine Synergistically Potentiates Mast Cell-Stabilizing Property of Ascorbic Acid. *Cell Physiol Biochem.* 2022;56(3):282-292. https://www.cellphysiolbiochem.com/Articles/000534/

181. USDA Agricultural Research Service. Accessed September 3, 2023. https://www.ars.usda.gov/

182. Cannataro R, Fazio A, La Torre C, Caroleo MC, Cione E. Polyphenols in the Mediterranean Diet: From Dietary Sources to microRNA Modulation. *Antioxidants.* 2021;10(2):328. doi:10.3390/antiox10020328

183. Ho CY, 한의혁, 채옥희, 김윤규, 김형태, 송창호. Scutellaria baicalensis Inhibits Mast Cell-Mediated Anaphylactic Reactions. *Anat Biol Anthropol.* 2010;23(4):217-227. http://journal.kci.go.kr/aba/archive/articleView?artiId=ART001509492

184. Roschek B, Fink RC, McMichael M, Alberte RS. Nettle extract (Urtica dioica) affects key receptors and enzymes associated with allergic rhinitis. *Phytother Res PTR*. 2009;23(7):920-926. doi:10.1002/ptr.2763

185. Zhang T, Finn DF, Barlow JW, Walsh JJ. Mast cell stabilisers. *Eur J Pharmacol*. 2016;778:158-168. doi:10.1016/j.ejphar.2015.05.071

186. Haftcheshmeh SM, Mirhafez SR, Abedi M, et al. Therapeutic potency of curcumin for allergic diseases: A focus on immunomodulatory actions. *Biomed Pharmacother*. 2022;154:113646. doi:10.1016/j.biopha.2022.113646

187. Maintz L, Novak N. Histamine and histamine intolerance. *Am J Clin Nutr*. 2007;85(5):1185-1196. doi:10.1093/ajcn/85.5.1185